THE HPV VACCINE CONTROVERSY

THE HPV VACCINE CONTROVERSY

Sex, Cancer, God, and Politics: A Guide for Parents, Women, Men, and Teenagers

Shobha S. Krishnan, M.D.

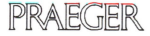

Westport, Connecticut
London

Library of Congress Cataloging-in-Publication Data

The HPV vaccine controversy : sex, cancer, god and politics : a guide for parents, women,
  men and teenagers / Shobha S. Krishnan.
      p. cm.
  Includes bibliographical references and index.
  ISBN 978–0–313–35011–5 (alk. paper)
1. Papillomavirus vaccines—Popular works. I. Title.
QR189.5.P36K75 2008
616.9′11—dc22   2008016056

British Library Cataloguing in Publication Data is available.

Library of Congress Catalog Card Number: 2008016056
ISBN: 978–0–313–35011–5

First published in 2008

Praeger Publishers, 88 Post Road West, Westport, CT 06881
An imprint of Greenwood Publishing Group, Inc.
www.praeger.com

Printed in the United States of America

The paper used in this book complies with the
Permanent Paper Standard issued by the National
Information Standards Organization (Z39.48–1984).

10 9 8 7 6 5 4 3 2

The author wishes to express that she is not sponsored by or affiliated with any
pharmaceutical company or commercial organization that promotes products related to the
subject matter of this book.

The contents and views presented in this book are for educational purposes only. No case-
specific medical advice will be provided. Please consult with your physician or a qualified
health-care professional for any personal questions or concerns.

*To my beloved husband, Mohan, and my wonderful
daughter, Anita*

CONTENTS

ACKNOWLEDGMENTS

This book would not have been possible without the help and support of

My patients, to whom I am deeply indebted for giving me their confidence and
trust, and from whom I have learned so much, and continue to do so.
All my mentors, particularly the late Dr. Irving Cohen, who have guided me
and shaped my professional career.

My special thanks to

Mathuram Santosham, MD, MPH: Director, Health Systems Program; Director,
Center for American Indian Health; Professor, Department of International
Health, Johns Hopkins University Bloomberg School of Public Health.
Michael P. McNeil, MS., Chair, Health Promotion Section, American College
Health Association and Assistant Director, Alice! Health Promotion, Health
Services at Columbia University.
Mary Commerford, Ph.D., Director, Furman Counseling Center, Barnard
College, Columbia University.
Brenda Slade, NP, MA, Director of Health Services, Barnard College, Columbia
University.
T. Rajkumar, M.D., D.M., Ph.D., Director and Professor, Department of
Molecular Oncology, Adyar Cancer Institute, Chennai, India.
Bernadette Stein, friend and fellow Trinity School parent, and Dan Stein, Dean
of Science, New York University.

Additional thanks are owed to

Debora Carvalko, Senior Acquisitions Editor, and her talented team at Praeger
Publishing for their wholehearted commitment to the project.
Stephanie Berger and Haylee Schwenk, for their prompt and superb editorial
counsel.
Zyamina Gorelik for her artistic insight.

Above all, I would like to thank my family for their love, encouragement, and moral support.

My sincere thanks to my brother-in-law, Chandra Sekar, M.D., a radiation oncologist in Parkersburg, West Virginia, for taking the time to read the entire manuscript. I deeply appreciate his sharing with me his vast experience in treating cervical and other HPV related cancers in the Appalachian population, where cancer rates are among the highest in the United States.

My deepest gratitude to my mother, Balam, for her enduring love and astute guidance, and in fondest memory of my beloved father, Swami Nath, who continues to be my greatest source of inspiration.

Lastly, my unwavering gratitude to my daughter, Anita, and my husband, Mohan, for their enormous patience, intense criticism, and keen sense of humor that helped me see this book to its fruition. I am glad that we are still an intact family!

Author's Note

Controversies, by their very nature, are difficult to discuss in reasonable terms. But a discussion can be especially hard when attitudes toward human sexuality, implications of science, and concerns over ethics collide. Such is the case with the new human papillomavirus (HPV) vaccine.

The controversy surrounding HPV vaccination pits the validity of science against moral and religious views. Proponents of the vaccine claim that it will provide unequivocal safeguards against a sexually transmitted virus that causes cervical cancer, but the vaccine has to be administered to girls between the ages of 11 and 12 in order to be fully effective. The decision whether to inoculate girls this young poses moral dilemmas to parents, religious leaders, and even some medical professionals, as they grapple with this polarizing issue. They find themselves asking the following question: should preteen children be vaccinated against a potentially cancer-causing sexually transmitted infection , or will the benefits of doing be outweighed by the potential for increased promiscuity and risky sexual behavior? Although these perceived risks of the vaccine may seem unfounded to those in the scientific community, many parents and religious leaders wonder whether the vaccine is just a "quick fix" to address the consequences of behavioral choices.

In spite of widespread opposition to the vaccine on moral and religious grounds, many states such as Texas proposed legislation requiring the vaccine to be administered to all young girls attending schools in those states. Several parents vehemently objected to the mandatory requirement of these shots. Furthermore, given that their preadolescent daughters' access to school hinges on a vaccine that is designed to prevent a sexually transmitted infection and that has to be administered even before the girls are old enough for their first school dance intensified their opposition. Many parents believe that there is a marked difference between mandating the vaccine for a disease that children get from casual exposure in a classroom, such as from coughing and sneezing, compared to contracting a disease that one acquires from "risky" personal behavior. Thus, the HPV vaccine poses a series of ethical dilemmas that cannot be easily dismissed.

In considering options to deal with any ethical dilemma, a variety of approaches may be employed to come to a logical decision. The doctrine of utilitarianism considers the rightness or the wrongness of a decision based on its consequences. Simply put, a utilitarian approach asks "what should a person do" and advocates a course of action that will do the greatest good for the greatest number of people. Therefore, in the case of the HPV vaccine, if a cost-benefit analysis study shows that the efficacy of the vaccine would be the most cost-effective method to drastically reduce cervical cancer in girls, a utilitarian would conclude that state-mandated vaccination of all 11–12-year-old girls may be the best course of action. To utilitarians, the desirable end of significantly reducing the occurrence of cervical cancer would justify the means of children's being vaccinated even against the wishes of their parents.

Principlism is another approach employed in clinical settings to make ethical decisions. This theory states that, even though the benefits of HPV vaccination would have a positive impact on society by bringing cervical cancer rates down substantially, mandating the vaccine would conflict with the principles of autonomy—the individual's right to choose. Principlists argue that mandates undermine the inherent worth of a person by depriving the individual of the right to choose. This is especially so with HPV, which is not an infection like measles or mumps that one contracts through casual exposure to fellow students, but a disease that is acquired primarily through sexual contact.

Yet another approach to decision-making used by ethicists is the principle of double effect (PDE). This method of arriving at ethical decisions seeks to evaluate the moral implication of an action that can produce both good and bad effects. The main difference between Principlists and those who subscribe to PDE is that the latter voice concerns about the moral and immoral uses of the vaccine. They ask the question, "When both good and bad consequences can arise from an action, should one abstain from doing the good in order to avoid the potential bad?" In the case of the HPV vaccine, those who adhere to the principle of double effect fear that administering the vaccine to girls before their sexual debut may promote a false sense of security and contribute to sexual promiscuity.

Finally, religious and cultural ethics must be considered in the HPV debate. Religious and cultural ethicists, though not opposed to advances in science and technology, have several moral objections to the HPV vaccine. They believe that because HPV is an infection that is acquired primarily due to lifestyle choices, a "virtuous woman" should have no need for such a vaccine. These morally based concerns will certainly play a vital role in determining whether this vaccine acquires widespread acceptance by parents and adolescents alike, both in the United States and around the world.

And while we ponder these ethical dilemmas, our society, along with several others, has generally seen a dramatic shift in the past 50 years in the social attitude of adolescent sexuality. Prior to the 1960s, girls were expected to "police" their sexual feelings. But, with the introduction of the birth control pills in the 1960s and 1970s, there has been a lessening of guilt and an increased acceptance of premarital sexual experimentation among both sexes. Today, three out of four adolescents are sexually active by the time they are 19 and according to *The New York Times* issue of March 12, 2008, one in four teenage girls in the United States has a sexually transmitted infection.

With the rapid advances in the medical sciences, it is critical that we have a citizenry that is scientifically literate. While much has been written about the HPV vaccine, it is difficult for the lay person to find an objective perspective on this topic. News reports and pharmaceutical advertisements have brought the HPV vaccine to the national consciousness. Advertisements for *Gardasil* showing children skateboarding, playing basketball and skipping rope and chanting "O-N-E L-E-S-S, I want to be one less, one less" have also introduced people to the HPV vaccine. However, there is a dearth of clear, accurate, and up-to-date information on the HPV vaccine, especially outside of scientific journals.

The aim of this book is to better acquaint you, the reader, to become well-informed and educated with the disease manifestations of HPV and the role of the new vaccines. And, even though the vaccines have shown to be highly effective, lifestyle changes are required to maximize their effectiveness. This book will address these issues and, although I do not claim to have the answers for all the tough questions, it is my hope that the readers of this book will be empowered to intelligently tackle the controversial issues that surface when sex, science, and the morals of society intersect.

This book is designed for parents, women, men, and teenagers. Because HPV vaccinations are recommended for preadolescents, it will inform parents of the various options to consider in choosing whether to have the HPV vaccine administered to their young daughters. This book also includes a discussion targeted at adult women of their possible eligibility for the vaccine as well as the information required to prevent HPV-related diseases. Men will learn that HPV is not a problem that solely affects women—they too are at risk and can suffer from the consequences of HPV infections. It is hoped this book will also be an invaluable resource to the high school and college-aged population, because this is the age group in which HPV infections peak. With special focus on this group, I have included a chapter with excerpts from a university town hall meeting that discusses the most frequently asked questions and concerns about HPV infections and the vaccine. In addition, a final chapter

has been included that highlights some of the personal stories and anec-
dotes of cervical cancer from women in developing countries and the
potential role these vaccines might play in preventing cervical cancer in
those parts of the world. It is my intent to bring a more human, less clinical perspective to the subject wherever possible.

This book can be used in several ways. My guess is that you will first
leaf through the pages, reading the chapter highlights and viewing the
illustrations. You may then choose to read the book "cover to cover" or
use it as a reference book. For the benefit of those who plan to use this
book as a reference, I have repeated important information in several
chapters and cross-referenced topics for greater detail.

When examining a controversial topic such as this, readers often
expect the author to provide them with a set of recommendations that fit
a clear and concise blueprint. My undertaking here, however, is to introduce you to all sides of the story, and to show you why they matter, and
how science fits into the fabric of human sexual behavior. I hope you find
this discussion helpful and that this book provides a basic understanding
of the medical issues that will enable you to participate in the scientific
and moral debates that are bound to ensue when vaccines for other sexually transmitted diseases such as HIV, chlamydia, and herpes are
unveiled in the near future—preadolescents will once again be the primary targets for these vaccines.

We are about to begin a journey that interweaves this labyrinth of
human nature, clinical medicine, bioethics, public health, and public policy. I hope that the path we take is an informative one and that you are
able to arrive at decisions that prove beneficial to you, the individuals in
your life, and society as a whole.

1

THE HPV VACCINE CONTROVERSY: SCIENCE VERSUS FAITH

Both doctors and patients want marvels in modern medicine to be simple, clear, and straightforward. Unfortunately, in a complex discipline such as medicine, the potential benefits and perils of new discoveries are seldom seen in black and white. When a new drug is introduced into the market, some welcome it with open arms while many others turn into skeptics. The HPV vaccine is no exception. The benefits of the vaccine are self-evident—according to most scientists, it will irrefutably reduce the occurrence of the second leading cause of cancer in women around the world. Normally, you would think that this kind of medical break-through would earn much fanfare and be accepted unequivocally. Not true. On the contrary, the advent of this vaccine for cancer prevention has fallen prey to cultural wars. The vaccine's release has been accompanied by a stormy scientific, moral, and political controversy, entrenched in passionate rhetoric and hidden agendas.

The Advisory Committee on Immunization Practices (ACIP), an arm of the Centers for Disease Control (CDC), voted unanimously to recommend the HPV vaccine to all 11- and 12-year-old girls in June 2006. Soon after, lawmakers in many states wanted to make the vaccine mandatory, in order to ensure early prevention of cervical cancer in girls who were not then sexually active. Scientists thought that vaccinating all preteen girls was premature, while conservative parents voiced that mandatory vaccination was immoral and compromised their family values. These varied opinions have led to vocalizations from a number of colorful personalities who have brought the controversy to life and highlighted its numerous pitfalls: the age at which it is recommended, the ethical dilemmas, corporate greed, and public outrage, all of which continue to shape this debate.

Generally, scientists, religious leaders, and politicians are wary of one another's motives. As with most scientific theories and postulations, from the motion of planets to the Theory of Evolution, the HPV vaccine represents yet another step in the history of resistance to new concepts in science, and particularly new vaccinations. This resistance has led to consistent clashes between science and ethics, with conflicts made worse by the fact that many people consider neither of these factors to automatically trump the other when making medical decisions. As Stephen Hall, the author of *Merchants of Immortality* puts it, "Ethics is too important to be left to scientists, and science is too important to be left to ethicists, politicians and other non-experts."

As with any controversy, both sides of the HPV vaccine story deserve equal attention. And, just like in any good debate, it is important to understand the facts before delving into the controversies surrounding them.

THE FACTS OF HPV

So, What Is HPV, Really?

HPV is the human papillomavirus. It is neither the same as HIV (human immunodeficiency virus) or HSV (herpes simplex virus), nor is it a new virus. There are more than 100 types of HPV. They have been around for generations. HPV can cause anything from warts on hands, feet, and the genital area to cancer of the head, neck, anal, penile, and cervical regions. Most HPV infections have no signs or symptoms. Therefore, many people are unaware that they are infected and can transmit the virus to a sex partner.

Who Gets HPV?

First and foremost, it is important to understand that anyone can get HPV infections, although some HPV infections require genital contact. There are mainly two broad categories of HPV infections. The first category causes warts—cauliflower-like lesions—to grow on the hands and feet and is spread by skin-to-skin contact. The transmission does not require sexual contact of any kind, and this type does not cause cancer. The second category of infection is caused by sexual contact (not necessarily intercourse) with a partner who is already infected with one or more types of the HPV, some of which can cause cancer. As with any sexually transmitted disease, the chances of getting infected with HPV increase with the number of sexual partners a person has. An infected carrier can live many years without any visible symptoms or illness but can potentially always be an active transmitter to a sexual partner.

How Common Is HPV?

According to the CDC, HPV is the most common sexually transmitted disease. Approximately 20 million people are currently infected with the virus in the United States (Myers et al. 2000). About 6.2 million Americans get a new genital HPV infection each year (Weinstock et al. 2004). It is estimated that at least 50 percent of sexually active men and women will acquire genital HPV infection at some point in their lives. Some studies even suggest that by age 50, over 80 percent of women will have acquired genital HPV infections (Myers et al. 2000). Most infections are transient and clear up on their own.

What Are the Consequences of Having HPV?

One of three results can occur from HPV infection:
First, it is possible to become a carrier of HPV and never show symptoms for the rest of your life. It can take weeks, months, or even years after you are exposed to HPV to show symptoms of genital warts or have an abnormal Pap smear. For this reason, it is impossible for most people to know when and from whom they contracted the virus. In most instances, HPV is a harmless infection that does not result in visible symptoms or health complications. HPV infections are most common in women and men in their twenties, and most infections clear spontaneously. However, even when infected people are not showing symptoms, they could still be capable of passing the virus on to their sexual partners. This is done without any knowledge of whether the virus could take a more aggressive form or what the consequences could be either to them or to their partners.

The second possible outcome involves developing warts on your hands, feet, and anogenital area (around the anus and in the genital area), that could be irritating, visually unpleasant, and embarrassing. These warts almost never develop into precancerous or cancerous lesions.

The third and the most serious outcome of an HPV infection is that it can lead to precancerous and cancerous lesions of the cervix, vulva, vagina, urethra, anus, penis, mouth, and throat. Of these diseases, cervical cancer is the most significant. Currently, FDA statistics show that there are about 500,000 cases of cervical cancer annually around the world, with 250,000 deaths due to this disease.

In addition, one cannot underestimate the emotional toll it can take on a person who contracts HPV. Emotions of guilt, shame, and anger, compounded with the fact that there is no permanent cure, can create significant psychological upheaval.

Is There a Cure for HPV If I Am Already Infected?

No. Unfortunately, like all other viral infections, such as the common cold virus or the herpes virus, there is no cure for HPV. The good news is that most HPV infections resolve by themselves.

Is HPV the Cause of All Cervical Cancers?

Ninety-nine percent of cervical cancer in women can be directly attributed to HPV (Walboomers 1999). The cause for the other 1 percent is unknown. However, it should be noted that, out of the existing 20 million cases of HPV infections, *very few* actually progress to cervical cancer (NIH 1996).

Is There an Approved Vaccine That Is Available to Us *Now*?

Yes, *Gardasil* (manufactured by Merck) was approved in June 2006 by the FDA. *Cervarix* (manufactured by GlaxoSmithKline [GSK]) is slated to enter the U.S. market in late 2008. The current vaccines do not protect against all strains of the virus, but are designed to prevent 70 percent of all cervical cancers. *Gardasil* also protects against 90 percent of genital warts. It is important to note that neither vaccine prevents other sexually transmitted diseases such as herpes, AIDS, or gonorrhea.

Who Should Get the Vaccine?

The ACIP arm of the CDC approved the vaccine, *Gardasil,* for all girls aged 11–12. The vaccine can be given as early as nine years of age, as well as to females between 13 and 26 years, even if one has already been sexually active. The other vaccine, *Cervarix,* has not yet been approved in the United States.

Are There Any "Absolute" Ways To Prevent HPV?

The answer to this is an emphatic *yes,* but it may not be practical or realistic. The only absolute way to prevent HPV is total abstinence by both partners prior to their meeting and commitment to sex with only each other from that point forward. This means both you and your current sexual partner must not have any other sexual partners for your entire lives. This method of prevention clearly has serious limitations for most people.

Are There Any Tests to Detect HPV Before It Leads to Cervical Cancer?

Yes. For sexually active women, routine Pap smears can detect abnormalities several years before they turn into cancer. Cervical cancer is normally a very slow-growing cancer, and it can take decades from the time you have an abnormal Pap smear to the time you actually get cancer.

Perhaps the above information has already convinced you that the only way to proceed from here regarding the vaccine is a decision between you and your or your child's doctor. However, factual information is not the only factor in making health decisions. In the case of HPV, there are conflicting business interests (drug companies), professional interests (doctors), religious interests (pastors and priests), political interests (politicians and community leaders), and last but not least, parents and teenagers. The topic of sex among teenagers has always been a political hotbed in the United States, creating the perfect recipe for controversy. These different groups have taken numerous steps to forward their agendas, and each group has been met with increasing opposition—with the various parties citing freedom of choice, freedom of speech, and even life, liberty, and the pursuit of happiness as justifications for their arguments.

The questions remain: Why do so many controversies surround the HPV vaccination? If each group claims they are acting in the best interest of women and teenagers, shouldn't we be in total agreement? The answer is yes—but even though each group wants to achieve the "big picture" of protecting women and teens, each sees the "correct" path to achieving this goal quite differently.

The Controversy: Different Viewpoints Regarding the HPV Vaccine

Proponents of the Vaccine

Proponents of the vaccine argue practicality over morality. Sure, most parents want their children to practice total abstinence until marriage. However, many parents realize that in a society where nearly 50 percent of girls and boys are sexually active before graduating from high school (CDC), total abstinence may not be a practical doctrine. Therefore, they are in agreement to take precautions to protect young women against possible repercussions of their sexual activity. After all, even if a young woman stays a virgin until marriage, the only way to guarantee that she will not contract HPV is if her spouse was also a virgin, no marital infidelity occurs, and the couple never divorces. In addition, most teens who do practice abstinence do not do so because they fear diseases like HPV. Therefore, a vaccine that eliminates the possibility of HPV will not eliminate their reason for abstaining from sex. For example, if fear were the seminal factor in determining celibacy and morality, the whole country would have been abstinent when the AIDS epidemic hit all cross-sections of society. However, research shows that fear of disease does not prevent sexual activity. Some factions even support the views stated in the article "Virginity or Death" in *The Nation* that holding back the vaccine is "honor killing on the installment plan." Likening the administration of the vaccine to providing a license to be promiscuous is similar to saying, in the words of Governor Perry of Texas, that a vaccine for lung cancer would strongly encourage smoking. Or, one could say that the safety devices in automobiles such as airbags, anti-lock brakes, and traction controls encourage us all to drive rashly and have more accidents. This argument discounts people's choice to exercise their own caution, common sense, or individual values and morals.

Another argument against the "increased promiscuity" hypothesis is that the HPV vaccine protects against only *one* of *many* sexually transmitted diseases. So, vaccination will not and should not preclude people from taking the usual and customary precautions for preventing other forms of sexually transmitted infections.

The next argument against the HPV vaccination states that the drug companies that have developed it have done so purely for profit and not in the best interest of consumers. However, one must accept that drug companies and medical researchers have done us a world of good with beneficial discoveries like penicillin and anesthetics. Developments like these have played a large part in making medical procedures—like undergoing surgeries, fighting infections, and even visiting the dentist—much more tolerable. It takes years of diligent and expensive research for the medical community to develop drugs that can be safely used by humans. Hence, drug companies must have the ability to continue to sell their drugs at a profit (within reasonable limits) in order to continue to do research to keep the human race healthy and functioning. Although vaccines can have inherent risks, they seem insignificant when compared to the good they have done for humanity.

Opponents of the Vaccine

Opposition to the vaccine is based on the premise that recognizing the possibility of teenage sexual activity endorses and encourages such behavior. Because HPV is a sexually transmitted infection, the vaccine has to be administered before girls begin engaging in sexual activity. Some people believe that girls who would have otherwise remained abstinent until marriage will be encouraged to become sexually promiscuous when they have been vaccinated against a sexually transmitted disease.

Another stance against mandatory HPV vaccination is that it constitutes unwarranted governmental intrusion. Because HPV is not spread by involuntary behavior like sneezing or coughing but rather voluntary, sexual behavior, some people believe that vaccination should be an individual or parental choice as opposed to a governmental one.

In addition, many uncertainties surrounding the vaccination still exist. While all the adverse reactions of the vaccine are still unknown, pharmaceutical companies are already making billions of dollars from advocating what some believe is an unnecessary vaccine. Dr. Bernard Carroll, a professor emeritus at Duke, calls such aggressive salesmanship "experimercial." He believes that an experimercial exists not to advance science but to increase the market share of a drug that has already been approved. This leads the public to wonder if medical professionals are working in the best interest of their patients. For example, doubters ask, if the purpose of the vaccine is really to prevent a common sexually transmitted disease, why are only women being vaccinated? Shouldn't men be a part of the equation? In addition, opponents of the vaccine believe that a pharmaceutical company like Merck may have an ulterior motive for promoting *Gardasil*. Reeling from the recall in 2004 of one of its most celebrated pain killers, *Vioxx*, Merck would be set to see a jump of up to $4 billion a year in profits if *Gardasil* were covered by private insurance plans and some government plans.

Moral and Political Backlash

The introduction of a vaccine to fight cervical cancer is an exciting advance in medical technology. However, the fact that the virus is transmitted through sexual contact is what has some conservative groups worried. These opponents of the vaccine say that a disease caused by possibly immoral behavior (having multiple sexual partners or partners outside of marriage) should be treated by ending that behavior as opposed to encouraging that very behavior by removing the medical repercussions. Several religious and moral groups believe that the HPV vaccine will contribute to the decay of our society's morals and values.

Tony Perkins, president of Family Research Council (FRC is a Christian organization promoting the traditional family unit and the Judeo-Christian value system as the basis for a just, free, and stable society), has said that the HPV vaccine sends the wrong message. "Our concern is that this vaccine will be marketed to a segment of the population that should be getting the message about abstinence," he said. Concerned Women for America (a U.S. coalition of conservative women that promotes Biblical values and family traditions) added, "It is the right and responsibility of parents—not government—to choose whether or not their daughters receive the vaccination." The same sentiments were shared by conservative parents across the country who echoed that the HPV vaccine would promote sex without consequences.

> ☞ **Opponents of the vaccine believe that vaccinating 11- and 12-year olds for a sexually transmitted disease will promote sexual promiscuity.**

Educate or Mandate?

Should HPV vaccines be mandated, or should parents and individuals decide? Mandate or choice has been debated many times over since the introduction of vaccines. This debate came up one more time in early 2007 when Rick Perry, the governor of Texas, tried to mandate the HPV vaccine for all girls between the ages of 11 and 12 within 8 months of its release. In a move that many parents and opponents of the vaccine saw as dictatorial, he issued an executive order mandating the vaccine, bypassing both public debate and the Texas legislature. Some people believe that mandates such as these are sound public health policies because they are the best way to assure that girls in underserved and socioeconomically deprived areas will be vaccinated. Proponents of mandatory vaccination argue that school dropout rates increase after age 13, so girls must be vaccinated before that age. Furthermore, statistics have shown that younger dropouts are more prone to engage in riskier sexual behavior. The hope is that when these children leave school, they will have already been vaccinated due to the mandate, thus making cervical cancer less likely in the next generation of underprivileged women.

> ☞ Proponents of the HPV vaccine believe that a mandate is a sound public health policy. They say it is the best way to assure that girls in socioeconomically deprived areas—where cancer rates are the highest—will be vaccinated.

In addition, some people believe that, instead of mandating the HPV vaccine, the government should spend money on sex education that promotes total abstinence. This situation puts the burden on the parents to educate their children and hold them to total abstinence, but we all have our own strong views about the pragmatism of such steps.

Financial Debate

Merck has heavily lobbied politicians and other institutions to mandate vaccination of teenage girls before entering middle school. Such aggressive lobbying caused some people to question if Merck was putting its business motives over the health of the people, absurd or unlikely as this may seem to others.

In addition, potential conflicts of interest exist between lobbyists and legislators. For example, the Texas Governor's former chief of staff, Mike Toomey, is Merck's key lobbyist in Texas. The current chief of staff's mother-in-law, Rep. Dianne White Delisi, is the state director for Women in Government, an association of state legislators that has organized fights against cervical cancer and has received funds from Merck, GSK, and Digene (a company that makes test kits to detect the presence of HPV). Their association blurred the motives of the Texas "mandate," and eventually, the house overrode Governor Perry's executive order requiring girls to get vaccinated before entering the sixth grade.

Finally, another question remains: Who will pay to vaccinate the young women who would receive the HPV vaccine? The vaccine requires a series of three shots each costing about $120 (excluding administrative costs). Will it be the government, the insurance companies, or the individuals who bear the brunt? If the financial burden falls on the state governments, it will stretch out the already taxed public health care system. Besides, it is not known at this time if booster shots will be required. In addition, with so much debate over mandating the vaccine, it seems possible that the public might not be willing to use tax dollars to pay for a vaccine for a sexually transmitted disease. Even vaccine advocates know that paying for mandatory vaccination would be a daunting task. If the vaccine were to be a national school requirement, approximately $900 million per year would have to be allocated for covering the female cohort of 2 million girls (2 million girls: $120 per dose plus a $25 administration fee for each of the three doses).

GlaxoSmithKline is the other pharmaceutical company that has developed an HPV vaccine, which is awaiting approval in the United States in the later part of 2008. Opponents who are skeptical of the vaccine requirement wonder if the current push to vaccinate is a strategy by Merck to be an incumbent before GSK releases its product into the U.S. market in the coming months.

LEGISLATIVE UPDATE

As of February 2008, various states have taken stands on the HPV vaccine. Other states are also preparing to address the HPV vaccine policy in their respective locales (see Table 1.1). For the latest updates on legislation regarding the vaccine, please refer to http://www.ncsl.org/programs/health/HPVvaccine.htm.

Table 1.1 HPV Vaccine: Introduced Legislation State by State

State	Summary	Status
Alaska	Requires offering a voluntary HPV vaccination program.	Passed
Arizona	Would fund outreach and education programs for the vaccine.	Pending
	Would require insurance companies to cover the cost of the HPV vaccine.	Pending
California	Would have required girls entering sixth grade to receive the vaccine.	Withdrawn
	Would require insurance companies that cover cervical screening programs to cover the cost of the HPV vaccine.	Pending

Colorado	Would require girls to receive the vaccine before entering sixth grade. Parents have the option to opt out. (The "opt-out" clause allows parents to refuse the vaccine for their children on medical, religious, or philosophical grounds.)	Postponed indefinitely
	Allocates 4% of state tobacco settlement money for cervical cancer education and immunization programs. Requires Medicaid and some health insurance companies to cover the cost of the vaccine.	Signed into law
Connecticut	Would require the first dose of the HPV vaccine to be administered to girls before entering sixth grade. Parents have the option to opt out.	Pending
	Would appropriate funds for HPV and cervical cancer programs and provide coverage for the vaccine through the state's insurance program.	Pending
District of Columbia	Would require girls to receive the vaccine before the age of 13.	Pending
	Parents have the right to opt out their daughters.	Pending
Florida	Would have required 11–12-year-old girls to receive the vaccine before entering sixth grade.	Died in committee
Georgia	Would mandate the vaccine for girls before entering sixth grade, unless parents give a written statement that they cannot afford it.	Pending
Hawaii	Would require Department of Health and Department of Education to educate parents about the link between HPV infections and cervical cancer.	Pending
	Would allow HPV to be added to the teen vaccination program and urge health insurance companies to cover the vaccine for females ages 11–26.	Pending

Illinois	Would require 11–12-year-old girls to receive the vaccine before entering sixth grade, with opt-out options for parents.	Pending
	Would require insurance companies to cover the vaccine. Would also require Department of Health to cover the vaccine for girls under the age of 18 who are not covered by an insurance provider.	Signed into law
Indiana	Would not mandate the vaccine. Instead, the Department of Health provides parents of sixth graders information about HPV and cervical cancer and asks them to sign a form about their decision to vaccinate or not. The school, in turn, must provide the information to the state health department.	Signed into law
Iowa	Would fund HPV and cervical cancer awareness programs. Also will have Department of Health cover the vaccine at no charge for females between the ages of 19 and 26 with incomes below 250 percent of federal poverty guidelines.	Pending
Kansas	Would require 11–12-year-old girls to receive the vaccine before entering sixth grade, with opt-out options for parents. Will also provide educational materials to parents about HPV and cervical cancer.	Pending
Kentucky	Would require 11–12-year-old girls to receive the vaccine before entering sixth grade, with opt-out options for parents. Would also provide educational materials to schools and the public about HPV and cervical cancer.	Referred to Senate
Maine	Vaccination is not required. Coverage provided through Maine Care program.	Signed into law
Maryland	Would require 11–12-year-old girls to receive the vaccine before entering sixth grade.	Withdrawn

Massachusetts	Would require 11–12-year-old girls to receive the vaccine before entering sixth grade, with opt-out options for parents. Would also provide for universal coverage of the vaccine.	Pending
Michigan	Would require 11–12-year-old girls to receive the vaccine before entering sixth grade. Parents should receive educational materials about the vaccine and be allowed to opt out their daughters if they so wish.	Pending
Missouri	Would require 11–12-year-old girls to receive the first shot before entering sixth grade. Parents will be provided educational materials but will be allowed to opt out their daughters by signing a form.	Pending
Minnesota	Would require girls entering sixth grade to be vaccinated. Opt-out provisions allowed.	Pending
	Created a study to closely review the risks, benefits, availability, efficacy, and coverage of HPV vaccine.	Signed into law
Mississippi	Would have required all sixth graders to be vaccinated. Financial questions and lack of opt-out clause cited as problems.	Died
Nebraska	Will first study the efficacy, funding, and the population covered by the vaccine.	Pending
Nevada	Requires health insurance companies to cover the vaccine for those who want it.	Signed into law
New Hampshire	Created a voluntary program which can provide the vaccine free to girls between the ages of 11–18 was created.	Passed and currently in force
New Jersey	Would require public education and distribution of information specific to the HPV vaccine to parents and guardians.	Signed into law
	Would require State Health Benefit Program, Medicaid, and New Jersey Family care to cover the cost of the vaccine.	Pending

New Mexico	Would mandate that girls between nine and 14 receive the vaccine. Provides opt-out clause for parents.	Vetoed
	Insurance plans in state to cover the vaccine for girls between nine and 14 years.	Signed into law
New York	Would require girls born after January 1, 1996 to be vaccinated. Provides opt-out clause for parents.	Pending
	Would require insurance companies that cover well-child visits and cervical screening programs to cover the vaccine for the 9–26-year age group. Passed a budget of $5 million to promote HPV vaccine.	Pending Signed into law
North Carolina	Requires Department of Health to provide educational materials to be distributed to parents of children in grade 5–12.	Signed into law
North Dakota	Requires information on HPV, its link to cervical cancer, and the role of the HPV vaccine to be distributed to the public.	Signed into law
Ohio	Would require all girls entering sixth grade to be vaccinated. Schools will not allow any student to attend classes for more than 14 days without written information on when they are receiving the vaccine, but parent opt-out options apply.	Pending
Oklahoma	Would require all girls entering sixth grade to be vaccinated. Opt-out provisions allowed.	Pending
Oregon	Would require health benefit plans to cover the HPV vaccine for girls 11 years and older.	Pending
Pennsylvania	Would designate January as cervical cancer awareness month and include HPV vaccine in the campaign. Would require health insurance companies to cover the cost of the vaccine.	Pending
Rhode Island	Would require health insurance companies to cover the cost of the vaccine.	Pending

State	Description	Status
South Carolina	Would require all girls entering sixth grade to be vaccinated. Opt-out provisions allowed.	Pending
South Dakota	Allocated $9.2 million in funds to the Department of Health to offer the HPV vaccine to women between the ages of 11 and 18.	Signed into law
Tennessee	Would require the Department of Health to provide information on the state of HPV infections in the various age groups, so that an appropriate policy for the vaccine can be established.	Pending
Texas	Governor issued an order to mandate vaccine in all girls entering sixth grade. Would distribute educational materials in both English and Spanish.	Vetoed by Texas legislature Pending
Utah	Established a cervical cancer awareness program	Signed into law
Vermont	Would require girls before entering sixth grade to be vaccinated. Opt-out provisions allowed.	Pending
Virginia	Requires girls 11 or older to receive the vaccine. Opt-out clause available.	Mandate to go into law effective 10/1/2008. Currently reconsidering the bill.
Washington	Provides all parents of sixth graders with information on HPV infections and where they can get the vaccine. Vaccination not required.	Signed into law
West Virginia	Would require girls before entering sixth grade to be vaccinated. Opt-out provisions allowed.	Pending

Source: Based on information from the National Conference of State Legislatures.

2

HPV Transmission and Natural History: A "Silent Epidemic"

Myth: All HPV infections cause symptoms.

Fact: HPV infections *rarely* cause symptoms. In most cases, they clear up on their own without causing any harm.

HPV Origins

The human papillomavirus (HPV), which comprises a group of more than 100 different viruses, has been in existence since time immemorial. The different HPV groups—also called types or strains—can cause a variety of infections, from benign warts on the hands and feet to cancer of the cervix, anus, penis, mouth, and throat. The word "papilloma" means an outwardly projecting finger-like growth that looks much like a cauliflower. The warts caused by HPV resemble papillomas; hence the name of the virus—human papillomavirus. These viruses are tiny, but one should not be fooled by their size alone; they are sturdy, extremely resilient, and very durable. It is anybody's guess as to how HPVs originated or where they came from, but a plausible explanation is that organisms, during one of their evolutionary mutations, went through rapid genetic restructuring that resulted in a set of defective genes, the accidental consequence of which resulted in the birth of the various types of HPV.

The existence of HPV has even been depicted in early fairy tales and folklores. Villainous characters with grotesque appearances and witches with unsightly extraneous bumps on their face and hands (which we now know as warts) were attributed to God's wrath on the immoral and evil sinners. One can only imagine how communities in those days regarded infected people as hideous and ostracized them because of the visible symptoms of this disease.

The study of germs and viruses has both fascinated and terrorized humans throughout the ages. Scientists have been studying viruses for a long time and are only too familiar with the natural tendency for viruses to mutate and multiply inside the human body. They have also observed that viruses adapt themselves like a predator to a prey in humans and adjust themselves to the rapidly changing host environment—to fulfill their self-serving mission of reproducing and transmitting themselves from one human to another. For example, we know that the common cold is caused by viruses. But to this day, there is no remedy because the cold viruses mutate rapidly to remain one step ahead of the scientists who are trying to find a method to eradicate them; it is no wonder that when patients go to their doctors with the common cold, the common joke is that it will take them one short week to cure the patients, but, if left untreated, it will take nature seven long days to get rid of it. It is for the same reason that the flu vaccine has to be reformulated annually in order to combat the waves of variant strains that sweep in each year.

Virology—the Study of Viruses

Scientists who were researching HPV observed one unique peculiarity of HPV strains—they were very "species" specific. This meant that the HPV species that grew on humans did not grow on cows (cows have their own strains of papillomavirus) and vice versa. This posed several challenges; HPVs were very difficult to grow on laboratory animals, and cross-infections did not occur. Thus, the researchers were not able to use the standard methods of conducting extensive research on animal test subjects to accelerate the finding of treatment and cure for this disease.

The bulk of our understanding of HPV today has been gained with the help of the electron microscope and advances in molecular biology, both of which have shed light on the structure of HPVs, how they affect humans, where they live, and how they carry out their functions and transmit themselves. There was one burning question for which scientists sought the answer: what makes the papillomaviruses so specific to one species or for that matter to specific sites? They found that each HPV type has a unique "key" on its surface that fits a complementary "lock" on a cell. So HPV types that cause warts on the hand can only attach themselves to the cells on the hand and not to cells in other parts of the body such as the cervix or the mouth. Due to this affinity of the different types of HPV for different sites on the body, it would be highly unlikely for someone to get warts in their genital area by merely shaking hands with someone who has a wart on his or her finger.

As HPV is very specific, each is given a strain or type number. For example, HPV types 1 and 2 most commonly cause warts on the hands and feet, types 6 and 11 cause genital warts, and types 16 and 18 cause precancerous and cancerous lesions of the cervix, vulva, vagina, penis, anus, mouth, and throat. These HPV type numbers were assigned to show the order of the virus strain discoveries (de Villiers et al. 2004).

Each HPV type has a protein covering called the capsid, and an interior made of two strands of DNA, the genetic material that is also made up of proteins. The DNA in any cell or virus is called its genome. The genome is *the* unique identifying signature of any living cell. Each and every living being is made up of billions of strands of DNA with each strand containing its unique genome. Each genome is broken down into smaller units called genes. The genes act like the memory or data banks for the genome, and they contain all the information that is needed for the HPV to reproduce. The HPV genome is no different functionally from the human genome, except that the HPV genome is much smaller. In fact, it may seem incredible that the two virulent strains of HPV, types 16 and 18, only have eight genes each (compared to humans who have several thousand), and these eight diminutive genes create all this havoc in the human race. Of all the HPV genes, there are two that are mainly responsible for the potential to cause cancer—the E6 and E7 genes. (The "E" designation indicates that these two genes are expressed early in the HPV life cycle.) These two genes invade the host cells (in this case humans), rearrange their genetic material, and inactivate the proteins that safeguard the cells. They also effectively render the defense mechanism of the host cell impotent and then proceed to use the host cell as their manufacturing plants to multiply in a highly disorganized fashion to form abnormal and mutated cells (Duensing et al. 2004). It is the accumulation of these abnormal cells that leads to warts and precancerous and cancerous cells. The more abnormal cells that form, the bigger the growth or lesions, and the more abnormal the cells are, the more severe the condition.

Along with the two cancer-causing genes, there is a third gene that has recently gained clinical significance: the L1 gene. This gene is important because it is responsible for the protein found on the viral capsid (or protein covering) on which the new vaccine technology is based—a topic covered in detail in Chapter 6 of this book.

INCIDENCE AND PREVALENCE

In epidemiology—the study of how diseases occur in different groups of people and why—the term "incidence" refers to the number of new occurrences of an infection or disease over a period of time (e.g., one year), and "prevalence" is the measure of the total number of infections or disease in a population at a given point in time. According to the Centers for Disease

☞ HPV is a silent epidemic. Fifty to 75 percent of HPV infections occur in women and men between the ages of 15 and 25 years.

Control (CDC), there are around 6.2 million new cases of HPV infections in the United States per year (incidence) and approximately 20 million people infected by the virus at any given time (prevalence). The greatest risk factors are age and sexual activity, with the highest rates being consistently found among sexually active men and women less than 25 years of age (Peyton et al. 2001); almost 50 to 75 percent of HPV infections are seen in men and women between the ages of 15 and 25 years. This is not surprising when one considers that this is the age group that practices the most risky sexual behaviors—unprotected sex, multiple partners, and high frequency of sexual activity. It is also estimated that about 80 percent of all sexually active men and women will acquire the infection at some point in their lives by age 50. Based on this knowledge, scientists have been able to make recommendations for the timing of cervical screening programs and the development of the vaccines to prevent HPV infection.

The occurrence of HPV infections is more common than most people think, but very few infections actually graduate all the way to cancer. The statistics tell the story: 70 percent of all infections clear within one year from the time they are contracted, and 90 percent clear within two years (Ho et al. 1998; Mosicki et al. 1998). The average duration of new infections is about eight months. Infections with the cancer-causing strains of HPV that persist beyond the normal duration are the most important factors in the development of invasive cancer. The time between initial HPV infection and development of cervical cancer usually takes *decades*. This is why the most common age at which one develops cervical cancer is around 35–50 years of age; the patient who develops cervical cancer at this age most probably got infected in their teen or early adult years.

According to the American Cancer Society, around 11,000 women develop cervical cancer and nearly 4,000 die from it annually in the United States. This burden is decidedly much greater worldwide. Globally, an estimated 500,000 new cases and 250,000 deaths occurred in the year 2000, with developing countries accounting for 85 percent of the cases and deaths from the disease. One can see that the disease exacts a tremendous toll on families and society as a whole year after year.

Human Papillomavirus Types and Their Disease Association

The HPV infection can manifest itself differently in various parts of the human body. It can occur externally or internally, cause benign or malignant lesions, and resolve on its own or develop into cancer.

As mentioned earlier, there are more than 100 types or strains of HPV. Of these 100 types, 60 cause warts on non-genital skin such as the hands and feet. These warts are called cutaneous warts (cutaneous means relating to the skin). Cutaneous warts are not caused by sexual contact and are widespread throughout the general population. Most of these warts are seen in school-aged children, especially those who are gymnasts and swimmers, due to increased warmth and moisture in these areas.

The other 40 types are called "mucosal" HPV. This means that they have an affinity for the body's mucous membranes, or the moist skin that is found in the oral, anal, and genital areas (Koutsky et al. 1999). These viruses do not prefer the skin on the hands and feet. Their transmission almost exclusively occurs through sexual activity, and therefore the diseases caused by them have been classified as sexually transmitted diseases.

The different HPV types can cause vastly different conditions in the various parts of the human body. The HPV strains and their various manifestations are illustrated in Figure 2.1

The common manifestations of HPV are covered in the following subsections.

Genital Warts

The HPV types that cause the infections leading to genital warts are known as "low-risk" viruses. Genital HPVs are normally accompanied by cauliflower-shaped warts on the anus and the genitals, also medically known as *condyloma acuminata*. These warts can occur internally in the anal and vaginal areas or can occur externally around the anus, the vagina, and the vulva. These warts do not progress to cancer. About 1 percent of HPV infections lead to genital warts. Ninety percent of genital warts are caused by HPV types 6 and 11 (Greer et al. 1995).

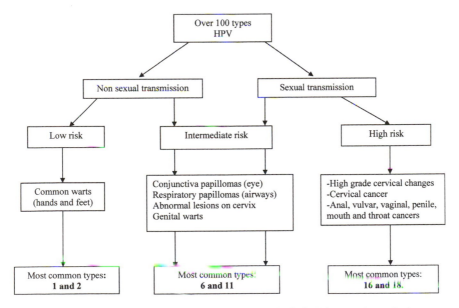

Figure 2.1 Human Papillomavirus Types and Their Disease Association

Abnormal Lesions of the Cervix (Dysplasias)

Abnormal lesions on the cervix are also called *"dysplasias"* (the word "plasia" means "growth" and "dysplasia" means "abnormal" growth). Cervical dysplasias can be mild, moderate, or severe. Severe dysplasia has the greatest tendency to progress to cancer. Cervical dysplasias can be caused by many types of HPV.

Cancer

HPV types that cause cancer are known as the "high-risk" viruses or oncogenic (cancer-causing) viruses (WHO 2000). The risk of persistence and progression to cancerous lesions varies by HPV type. The HPV 16 strain is the most common cancer-causing virus when compared to other types of HPV. HPV 16 alone is linked to more than 50 percent of all cervical cancers worldwide, followed by HPV 18, which is responsible for another 15–20 percent of all cervical cancers. These two types account for the majority of cases, 70 percent (Bosch et al. 2003), while the remaining 30 percent is caused by less common strains.

LIFE CYCLE OF HPV—NATURAL HISTORY

Natural history helps us understand the interrelationships of the organisms to their host environment. Before we embark on understanding the life cycle of the HPV in humans, it is best to review the anatomy of the female reproductive tract and gain a better understanding of what is normal and what is not. The emphasis here will be on the cervix, where the HPV predominately likes to reside.

The Female Genital Tract

Vulva

The vulva (not shown in the illustration) includes the labia majora (large lips) and labia minora (small lips). The labia majora is the area that is covered with hair after puberty. The labia minora is hairless and is made up of mucus membrane.

Vagina

The vagina is a cavity that forms the sidewalls of the cervix. It is the organ that accommodates the male penis during sexual intercourse, and it is also the organ that expands to become the birth canal.

Uterus

Also known as the womb, the uterus serves as a safe boarding place for the growing fetus. It nourishes and protects the fetus until delivery, when it is ready to make its entry into this world during childbirth.

Fallopian Tubes

These are two tubes that emerge from either side of the top of the uterus. These are the crucial passageways for sperm to travel to fertilize the egg. Once the egg is fertilized here, it travels to the uterus, embeds itself, and starts to grow.

Ovaries

The ovaries (not shown in the illustration) are the oval-shaped organs present at the end of the fallopian tubes. The ovaries house all the eggs; a female is born with all the eggs she can produce. In other words, what a woman is born with is what she will have—no more, no less. Each ovary takes a turn every other month to release an egg into the fallopian tube for potential fertilization.

Cervix

The cervix is the opening of the uterus. Its outer surface, the ectocervix (also called the exocervix), has an opening called the *os,* which dilates during childbirth. The cells on the ectocervix are made up of large, flat, hexagonal multilayered squamous cells (see Figure 2.2). The cells at the very top of this layer contain a material called keratin, which makes them hard. Keratin serves as a shield against foreign invasion of bacteria, viruses, and other unwanted organisms.

The inner surface of the cervix or the endocervix is connected to the uterus by a tunnel called the endocervical canal or the canal of the cervix. The endocervical canal is lined by tall columnar cells, also called glandular cells. These cells, unlike the squamous cells of the ectocervix, do not produce keratin, and therefore are more vulnerable to foreign invasion by bacteria and viruses. The region where the flat squamous cells of the ectocervix overlap the tall columnar epithelium of the endocervix is

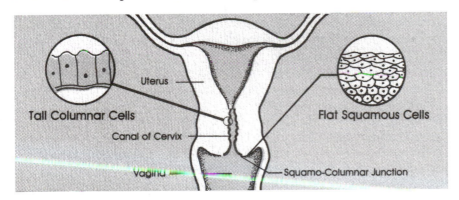

Figure 2.2 The Female Genital Tract
Source: Courtesy of Paul Indman, M.D.

called the squamo-columnar junction or the transformation zone (TZ). As you will soon see, the TZ is of particular interest to us because this is the area where the HPV prefers to infect the cells.

HPV Reproduction—Conquer and Divide

In many ways, human papillomaviruses are akin to a terrorist group. They have highly specific targets, thrive by destroying human cells, are hard to detect, and constantly carry out covert guerilla operations. Their dedication to their mission and goal of reaching the intended target site is remarkably unwavering. As mentioned earlier, depending on the strain of HPV, they can attack cells in any number of locations in the human body. However, they have a particular affinity for the squamous epithelial cells that line the outside and inside of several organs of the human body such as the mouth, throat, cervix, vagina, vulva, anus, and penis.

In order to understand the functions of HPV, one has to understand the basic fundamentals of the largest organ in the human body—the skin. The skin is made up of multiple layers of cells. The innermost or deepest layer is called the basal layer, and its sole purpose is to function as the manufacturing factory for the skin. The cells in the basal layer multiply and migrate to the surface to replace the dead cells that are shed by humans daily. During the migration process, they mature, change shape, and develop keratin, which hardens and acts as an additional protective layer for the skin. The cells on the surface of the skin constantly die as part of the normal physiological process, but the basal layer never does; it is almost immortal. The HPV takes advantage of this very characteristic by using the basal layer as its manufacturing factory and maintaining a reserve for itself there.

To infiltrate the basal layer, the virus first has to penetrate through several layers of skin. This skin penetration occurs when the outer layer is weakened by repeated trauma like that experienced during vaginal or anal intercourse. The more the skin is traumatized, the easier it is for the HPV to journey to the basal layer. When the opportunity strikes, the virus attacks the basal cell and mutates the DNA of the host cell to reflect that of the HPV. Now, when the mutated cell divides and multiplies, it is actually reproducing cells with the HPV DNA in them. These new HPV cells then follow the normal pattern of migration to the surface.

The only difference between the HPV cell and the normal cell is that, whereas the normal cell matures and dies at the surface, the HPV cells multiply rapidly, and they either do absolutely nothing or form warts or abnormal lesions. Eventually the HPVs transmit themselves from one person to another by exploiting a common human behavior—namely, sexual activity. The HPV cells' cycle of birth, migration, and rapid multiplication now continues in the new host. The entire reproductive cycle starts all over again.

The Teenage Cervix: What Makes Young Women So Vulnerable to HPV

What comes next is one of my favorite factoids in medicine that I always like to share with my adolescent patients. As I hope you will see, this is one of the most compelling scientific reasons for teens to delay sexual activity. Unfortunately, this pearl of wisdom is most often ignored and much less heeded than it should be.

As I mentioned earlier, in the cervix, the TZ or the squamo-columnar junction is the zone where the squamous cells of the ectocervix meet the glandular cells of the endocervix. This is one of the most vulnerable areas for infection by HPV and other invading micro-organisms (see Figure 2.2). During the course of a woman's life, the location of the TZ changes: at puberty, the TZ is wide and exposed on the ectocervix. As a woman reaches late adolescence and beyond (18–20 years), the squamous cells of the ectocervix undergo gradual keratinization, which provides better protection against infections. In addition, the TZ shrinks

> ☞ The teenage cervix is most vulnerable to HPV and other sexually transmitted diseases.

and retracts inside the cervical canal, thereby reducing the chances of infection. This is one of the main reasons young adolescent women are especially more susceptible to infections by HPV and other sexually transmitted infections.

TRANSMISSION

HPV is a modest virus. It attracts no attention to itself. It remains silent for weeks, months, and years and yet transmits itself freely. Silent infections are more the norm than the exception. An infected person, without ever experiencing any of the outward manifestations, is still capable of carrying and transmitting the virus under these circumstances to his or her sexual partner. For this reason, the transmission rates are very high and most HPV infections go unrecognized, thus rendering HPV a "silent epidemic."

All infectious diseases rely on transmission, or the spread of micro-organisms, for the onset of infection. HPV is predominantly transmitted through sexual activity (Winer et al. 2003). Even though sexual intercourse is the usual route of transmission, HPV can also be spread by many nonsexual routes. HPV can transmit itself skin to skin, skin to mucosal, mucosal to skin, or mucosal to mucosal membranes. Therefore, the transmission mechanisms conducive for HPV can be classified under two predominant types of activities—sexual and nonsexual—and are described in more detail later in this chapter and in Table 2.1. Unlike

HIV (human immunodeficiency virus), HPV is not transmitted through the blood or organ transplants.

HPV Transmission by Sexual Activity

The sexual activities in which humans generally partake can all contribute to the transmission of HPV between partners. The activities can be described as those involving intercourse—vaginal or anal—or contact without intercourse—oral sex and nonpenetrative sex such as foreplay.

Vaginal or Anal Intercourse

Most, if not all, infections occur through direct vaginal or anal intercourse (Winer et al. 2003). Transmission is thought to occur through mechanical abrasion of infected skin or a mucous membrane with uninfected skin or a mucous membrane. The minor or microscopic trauma caused to the epithelium during sex allows the HPV to cut through several superficial outer skin layers and gain entrance to the bottom basal cell layer where it likes to reside.

In Women

HPV is a common infection in women. More than 50 percent of college-age women are found to have an HPV infection within four years of their first sexual intercourse. Transmission of HPV cannot be prevented by urinating, washing the genitalia, or douching after sex.

In HIV-Positive People

Men and women who are HIV positive have a greater risk of HPV-related diseases than the general population. In addition, men who have sex with men and engage in receptive anal sex carry a higher risk of HPV infections and transmissions than others.

In Men

The transmission of the virus in men is still not well understood. It is believed that the infection in males is very short-lived and largely asymptomatic. There is now enough evidence to show that uncircumcised men are more likely to harbor the virus than circumcised men and that circumcision can actually lower the risk of HPV transmission and infection.

Condoms and HPV Transmission

Condoms are usually highly effective in reducing the transmission of sexually transmitted infections (STIs) that are transmitted through fluid discharge, such as HIV, gonorrhea, and chlamydia. For STIs such as HPV that are spread by skin-to-skin contact, condoms can still offer very good protection. Recent studies show that consistent and correct use of condoms can still significantly reduce the risk of transmission of HPV (Winer et al. 2006). So, even though the degree of protection may be lower, "thumbs up" to the proper use of condoms.

Female condoms have an even greater advantage over male condoms, in that their size and shape enable them to cover a wider surface area of the external genitalia that is normally not covered by the male condom. The downside to female condoms is that they are less affordable and less popular than male condoms.

Sexual Contact without Intercourse

Even though HPV transmission by nonpenetrative genital contact is rare (Winer et al. 2003), HPV infections have been detected in women who said that they did not have penetrative sex.

Nonpenetrative Sex
In nonpenetrative sex such as abrasive foreplay, HPV can be transmitted from the infected area of one partner to the uninfected area of another partner via skin-to-skin contact, skin-to–mucous membrane contact, or any combination thereof.

Oral Sex
In oral sex, HPV can spread from an infected genitalia to the oral cavity of the partner and give rise to oral warts, precancerous lesions, and cancer of the mouth. Transmission can also take place the other way around: that is, from an infected oral cavity to the genitalia. Fortunately, such occurrences are very rare.

HPV Transmission by Nonsexual Methods

Maternal

Although transmission from mother to the newborn child is relatively rare (Watts et al. 1998), the state of pregnancy weakens the immune system. In medical parlance, this is called an immunocompromised state. The hormonal changes caused by pregnancy can actually flare a subclinical or dormant condition of HPV in the mother into a full-blown disease. Mothers can pass on the virus to their babies during childbirth, and some strains can lead to considerable negative impact on the health and quality of life of the child. This is particularly true of a vaginal delivery where the baby passes through the birth canal that is infected with HPV with or without the mother's knowledge. HPV transmission from mother to child can cause:

Conjunctival Papillomas
The conjunctiva is the part of the eye where the inner eyelid and the eyeball meet. Warts may develop in these areas in infants and children. In order to relieve symptoms, the warts have to be removed. HPV types 6, 11, and 16 are frequently associated with this condition.

Respiratory Papillomatosis
Children can also develop warts in their airways that usually cause noisy breathing called *stridor*. About one in 200,000 children under the

age of 18 and mostly under the age of four develops respiratory papillomas. Unfortunately, in spite of removing the warts, they are strongly recurrent, and most grow back. HPV types 6 and 11 are frequently associated with this condition (Reeves et al. 2003).

Anal and Genital Warts

Anal and genital warts, though very rare, can be caused as a result of maternal transmission. It should be strongly emphasized, however, that the majority of cases of children who develop anal and genital warts are primarily a result of child molestation.

Cutaneous

This refers to nongenital skin-to-skin or skin-to-surface contact. Close personal contact is believed to be an important feature in HPV transmission, but it is not always necessary for the virus to spread. Children who participate in activities that take place in a warm, moist environment, such as swimming or gymnastics, and walk barefoot are particularly prone to getting warts called plantar warts on their feet. Warts are also common on the hands of children, members of crew teams, and butchers and meat handlers who invariably have minor cuts on their hands. HPV types 1 and 2 are commonly associated with cutaneous transmissions.

Autoinoculation

The dictionary defines autoinoculation as the process by which one infects or inoculates "a healthy part with an infective agent from a diseased part of the same body." An example of autoinoculation would be for a person who has warts on the vulva to transmit the virus to the anal region by either scratching the infected area or by inadvertently making contact with both areas during one's daily activities, such as using a towel in an infected area of the body and immediately making contact with a healthy area. The operating word here is *immediately*, as HPV cannot survive outside the living cell for very long.

Fomites

Fomites are inanimate objects that absorb, hold, and carry disease-causing germs that spread infections. Even though there are anecdotal references to HPV being spread by underwear and swim suits, their spread by fomites remains highly debatable and is rare (Frega et al 2003). For example, a study to see if HPV was spread through floors and seats of humid dwellings showed that it was highly unlikely (Puranen et al. 1996). Similarly, HPV cannot spread through contact with toilet seats, eating utensils, doorknobs, hot tubs, or bath tubs.

Table 2.1 Likelihood of HPV Transmission

Mode of Transmission	Likelihood of Infection
Unprotected vaginal intercourse—giving or receiving	Very high
Unprotected anal intercourse—giving or receiving	Very high
Oral sex	Possible
Foreplay	Possible
Protected vaginal intercourse—giving or receiving	Possible
Protected anal intercourse—giving or receiving	Possible
Towels	Possible—If rubbed from an infected genital area to an uninfected genital area *immediately*
Sex toys	Possible
Sharing, cups, glasses and spoons	Rare
Maternal	Can occur but rare
Swimming pools	Can get warts on feet from walking barefoot, but not genital warts.
Gym	Warts on hands and feet possible, but not genital warts
Sharing swim suits	Highly unlikely
Shaking hands with a person with warts	Possible—Can get warts on your hands, but not genitals.
Beds	No
Pets	No
Toilet seats	Highly unlikely
Sneezing	Never

A summary of the detailed discussion in this chapter is provided as a list of key facts for your quick reference.

Key Facts

- HPV is the most common sexually transmitted disease. About 20 million men and women in the United States have HPV infections, and about 6.2 million new cases occur each year.
- Nearly three out of four Americans between the ages of 15 and 49 have been infected with genital HPV.
- Sexual transmission is the most common mode of transmission. There are over 100 types of HPV, out of which 40 types are transmitted sexually and cause genital HPV infections and diseases. A little more than a dozen of these are cancer-causing viruses.
- HPV is a silent disease. HPV can be contracted through a partner, remain dormant, and be transmitted to the next partner without symptoms.
- Genital HPV can also spread through skin-to-skin contact.
- Most HPV infections resolve spontaneously and rarely lead to cancer.

3

RISK FACTORS AND TESTING: KNOWLEDGE IS POWER

Myth: Promiscuity is the main reason people get HPV infections and, therefore, cervical cancer.

Fact: One can get an HPV infection even from a monogamous relationship. Several other factors come into play to cause HPV infections to lead to cancer.

The human papillomavirus has been around for centuries, but it still remains an enigma. HPV infections run very unpredictable courses, ranging from harmlessly resolving on their own to causing debilitating cancers. It is important to understand that while HPV infections are necessary to cause most cervical cancers, they *alone* are not sufficient to cause the disease (Bosch et al. 2003). So, what are the other factors that, in conjunction with HPV, influence the risk of progression from infection to cancer? There are several risk factors that work in close partnership with HPV infections to cause more serious types of HPV-related diseases.

> **HPV infections are necessary, but not solely sufficient, to cause cervical cancers or other HPV-related diseases.**

A risk factor is any condition that increases your chances of getting a disease. For example, diabetes is a risk factor for heart disease. Smoking is a risk factor for lung cancer. And in this case, HPV is a risk factor for cervical cancer. Risk factors increase your odds of getting the infection or the disease but by no means are a guarantee that you will get the disease. As always, one can develop cancer without any of the known risk factors. Risk factors for HPV infections fall into two broad categories—ones that "fire" infections and those that "fuel the fire." Risk factors that fire HPV infections are activities that help a person contract HPV infections in the first place, such as having sex with multiple partners and having unprotected sex. Risk factors that fuel the fire have the potential to act as catalysts and propel HPV infections to progress to precancerous and cancerous lesions.

Risk Factors That "Fire" the Infection

The single, most significant risk factor that increases your chances of acquiring an HPV infection is your sexual behavior.

Early Age at First Intercourse

The younger the age of first intercourse, the more likely a person is to be exposed to HPV and other STIs. There are several reasons for this: The transformation zone (TZ; refer to Chapter 2 for a more detailed discussion) is larger and more exposed to infections in teenage girls. This, coupled with other high-risk behaviors such as smoking and unprotected sex, makes teens more vulnerable to HPV and other sexually transmitted infections (ACS).

History of Having Multiple Sexual Partners

This is basic math: The more sexual partners you have, the more likely your chance of contracting the virus. For example, commercial sex workers with exceedingly high numbers of sexual partners have a very high risk of cervical cancer, while celibate women such as nuns have a very low risk. In virtually all studies, the most consistent predictor of HPV infection was the number of sex partners (Manhart et al. 2006; Trottier & Franco 2006). That does *not* mean that women who get cervical cancer are promiscuous. For example, if your partner has a cancer-causing strain of HPV and he or she is the only person you have had sexual contact with, then that will increase your risk of getting this high-risk strain.

Having a Sexual Relationship with a Partner Who Has Had Multiple Partners

There is a common saying: "If you are having sex with someone, then you are having sex with everyone that person has had sex with." This means that your chance of contracting HPV is also strongly dependent on your partner's prior sexual history (Winer et al. 2003)—in other words, the more partners, the higher the chance that one of you is infected and, consequently, the higher the chance of contracting or transmitting the infection, respectively. However, if you contract HPV from your current partner, this does not automatically mean that he or she is currently cheating on you: he or she could have contracted it from a past sexual encounter before meeting you.

Sexual Contact with a Partner Who Is Infected

If you are having sexual contact with an infected partner, then the chances of your getting HPV are very high.

Frequency of Sexual Intercourse

The more frequent the sexual intercourse with an infected partner, the higher the chance of the virus gaining access into your body.

Unprotected Vaginal or Anal Intercourse

This is the most common method for HPV transmission. It has been shown that condoms can significantly reduce the risk of HPV transmission.

Protected Vaginal or Anal Intercourse

No barrier methods can completely protect against HPV transmission because HPV is primarily transmitted through skin-to-skin contact. The virus can reside anywhere from the base of the penis to around the anus to any part of the pubic area. Therefore, in spite of using condoms, one can still get HPV from contact with the areas that are not covered by the condom. As discussed

 The most significant risk factor to acquiring an HPV infection is sexual behavior.

earlier, the only way to avoid HPV is to stay away from all genital to genital contact—not a viable option for most human beings.

RISK FACTORS THAT "ADD FUEL TO THE FIRE"

The following are risk factors that have the potential to act as catalysts and propel HPV infections to progress to precancerous and cancerous lesions.

A Weakened Immune System

A weakened immune system signifies the inability of the host's defense system to clear or resolve the HPV infection. This weakened condition helps you to acquire and retain the virus in your body, and it renders you unable to spontaneously stave off HPV infections. This allows for a longer duration of the infection and increases the likelihood of the persistence of the cancer-causing strains. The longer an HPV infection persists, the less likely a patient is to clear the infection (Ho et al. 1998). Some of the biggest culprits that contribute to weakening the immune system are outlined here.

Stress

Stress releases two hormones in our body, adrenaline and cortisol. These hormones, over time, suppress the immune system. This can weaken the body's natural defenses and allow infections like HPV to take the upper hand. For example, one man had been under a lot of stress with a new job—he had been traveling a lot and had gotten very little rest. One day his wife noticed "cauliflower-like" bumps on his penis, and his doctor confirmed their suspicion that it was HPV. One explanation the doctor offered the couple was that the virus may have been contracted from a past sexual partner and then lay dormant in his body for several years. His current condition of extreme physical and emotional stress had weakened his immune system and rekindled the virus.

Medications

Medications such as steroids, which are given for chronic diseases like rheumatoid arthritis, as part of cancer treatment, and after organ transplants, suppress the immune system and facilitate the persistence of HPV infections. The hormonal drug DES (Diethylstilbestrol), which was prescribed to pregnant women prone to having miscarriages in the 1940s through the 1970s, may also have been a strong risk factor. According to the American Cancer Society, one in 1,000 "DES daughters" (women whose mothers took DES) developed cervical cancer. It was observed that the incidence of cervical cancer was highest in those DES daughters whose mothers took the medication during the first 16 weeks of their pregnancy. However, one does not have to worry about being exposed to this drug any more, as it is no longer available in the United States.

HIV Infection

HIV damages the body's immune system. Hence, cervical and anal cancers are more common in people who are infected with the HIV virus. HIV also increases the rate at which precancerous lesions progress to cancerous ones.

Substance Abuse

Heavy drinking and substance abuse affect the body in a negative way both directly and indirectly. Directly, they can attack the DNA of the host cells and weaken the immune system. Indirectly, they can affect one's mental balance and affect sense of judgment. Drugs and alcohol are known to be major reasons for individuals indulging in high-risk behavior: having sexual encounters with strangers, having sex without protection, and encountering sexual assault. These behaviors not only increase one's risk of exposure to HPV but also to other sexually transmitted diseases like HIV, gonorrhea, and chlamydia.

Increasing Age

The younger you are, the higher the chances of acquiring and clearing HPV infections. The opposite is true as you get older (30 and above); the chances of being infected are lower, but, unfortunately, so are the chances of clearing the infection spontaneously. In addition, when you get HPV infections at an older age, they are more likely to be persistent and progress to a more serious condition. This is one reason there are more HPV infections in the younger population and more cervical cancer as one gets older. More than half of cervical cancer deaths occur in women over the age of 55. Loss of immunity during menopause can also increase the incidence of infection.

Poor Diet

Since the time of Hippocrates, health-care providers have understood the importance of diet and nutrition to patients' good health and well-being. Numerous studies have found that several nutritional factors, particularly a diet that is rich in fruits and vegetables (especially the green leafy varieties), are essential to ward off any illnesses or infections. On the other hand, a deficiency in antioxidants such as vitamins A, C, and E and a deficiency in folic acid have been found to weaken the immune system, cause cell damage, and promote the growth of abnormal cells. In order to offset this to some extent, a dietary supplement of one multivitamin a day is now recommended for people of all age groups. Regular exercise and maintaining ideal body weight also help people to stay healthy and boost their immune systems.

Pregnancy and Women with Many Children

In addition to all the other changes that their bodies go through, pregnant women are unfortunately more prone to the temporary weakening of their immune systems. Hence, there may be a reactivation of an already existing infection.

Women who have had many children and have gone through full-term pregnancies have a direct correlation to an increased risk of cervical cancer (Muñoz et al. 2002). Research has shown that women with three or more children are at a greater risk for cervical cancer than women with one or two children. Having the first baby before the age of 17 doubles the risk, compared to having your first baby at age 25.

Poor nutrition, repeated trauma, a weakened immune system, and hormonal changes can all influence the risk of persistence and progression of HPV infections.

Presence of Other Sexually Transmitted Diseases

Chlamydia is a sexually transmitted disease that infects the reproductive tract of women. It causes inflammation of the cervical lining and makes the cervix more vulnerable to HPV-induced abnormal changes (Samoff et al. 2005). It has also been found that the risk of HPV-related diseases are higher among women who have had three or more other STIs; it can be surmised that, perhaps, multiple STIs reduce the local immune responses and render women more susceptible to HPV. Another factor that could play a role is that women with three or more STIs may have had multiple sex partners, which also increases their risk for HPV infections.

Smoking

Here is one more excellent reason not to smoke. Smoking increases the risk of cervical cancer—and the evidence is compelling. Even though smoking by itself can contribute to less than 1 percent of cervical cancers (with 99 percent of cervical cancers being caused by high-risk HPV), it has been found that the combination of cigarette smoking and HPV infection dramatically increases one's chance of getting cervical cancer. One of the most notable researchers in this field has been Anthony Gunnell, a medical biostatistician and epidemiologist, and his colleagues in Stockholm. They conducted a large study comprising 105,760 women from 1969 to 1995 to address the potential interaction between smoking and HPV 16 (the strain that causes over 50 percent of cervical cancers) in the development of severe cervical dysplasia, which, if left untreated, is a precursor to cervical cancer. The findings of the study are as follows:

- Women who smoked and who were positive for HPV 16 were fourteen times more likely to get cervical cancer than women who smoked but were negative for HPV 16.
- Women who did not smoke and were positive for HPV 16 only had a sixfold increase in risk of cervical cancer when compared to women who did not smoke and were negative for HPV 16.

These findings are summarized in Table 3.1.

From Table 3.1 one can draw the conclusion that the detrimental factor that contributed to the jump from the baseline risk of 6:1 to 14:1 between the HPV-16–positive and HPV-16–negative women in the group was *smoking*—indicating that smoking was a contributory risk factor for the development of cervical cancer, in the presence of high-risk HPV infections.

Another study showed that the association of HPV and smoking was greater in current smokers versus former smokers, in heavier smokers

Table 3.1 Risk of Developing Severe Cervical Dysplasia as Found by Gunnell and Colleagues

Status	HPV 16 positive	HPV 16 negative	HPV 16 +/HPV 16 – ratio
Smoker	14	1	14:1
Nonsmoker	6	1	6:1

(10 or more cigarettes per day) versus lighter smokers, and as the number of pack years smoked increased (Harris et al. 2003). The highest risk of cervical cancer was found among women who smoked for at least five years and were positive for HPV 16 infection at the time of their first Pap smear, as compared to those who had smoked for a long duration but were HPV negative (Gunnell et al. 2006). Research also shows that passive smoke could be a risk factor for HPV-related cervical diseases (Coker et al. 2002).

These statistics show that the interaction between smoking and HPV-related diseases is of vital importance to public health, as most young men and women start smoking around the same age that they become sexually active, which is also when they are most prone to HPV infections. Based on observations of smoking related to risk of cervical dysplasias, it only makes sense to carefully monitor smokers who are positive for HPV. For their own improved health and wellness, they should also be strongly encouraged to quit smoking.

Now that it is clear that smoking increases the risk of cervical cancer, the questions are "how and why?" There are several possible reasons, some of them being: nicotine and tobacco-specific carcinogens such as benzyrene have been detected in the cervical mucus of smokers. These toxins damage the cervical cells and promote abnormal cell growth.

In addition, there is significant association between smoking, the persistence of HPV infections, and the development of related cervical lesions. It is believed that smoking weakens the local immunity and allows HPV infections to persist. This facilitates the development of abnormal cervical lesions (Barton et al 1998). Some studies have also shown that the cessation of smoking may actually help in the regression of minor grade lesions (Szarewski et al. 1996; Trimble et al. 2005). So, the message from all these studies is to *quit smoking.*

> ☞ **Smoking is a major risk factor for HPV-related disease.**

The Pill

For most women, the biggest worry about having sex is not about acquiring an STI but about getting pregnant. So when they choose the pill as their form of contraception, many stop using condoms as a precaution and, thus, expose themselves to HPV infections and other STIs. Studies have shown that there is an association between the pill and HPV. However, it is important to note that the increase in the rate of HPV infections from the pill is small. Women who start the pill at age 20 or younger and women who have taken the pill for more than five years may also be at a higher risk of having persistent HPV.

Women who start the pill at age 20 or younger have an increased risk for cervical cancer when compared to those who started taking the pill after the age of 20 (Moreno et al. 2002). Whether this is directly related to oral contraceptives (OCs) is not known. A possible explanation is that women who began taking OCs before the age of 20 probably initiated sex at a younger age. As discussed earlier, teens have a wide and exposed TZ that makes them much more prone to HPV and other STIs at this young age. Also, many may have multiple sexual partners and engage in more risky behaviors, which may compound the risk associated with OCs.

The scientists at the National Cancer Institute and the International Agency for Research on Cancer (IARC) have also shown a relationship between the extended use of the pill (beyond 5 years) and a slight increase in the risk of cervical cancer. However, it has not yet been determined if the prolonged use of OCs is an independent risk factor for cervical cancer. As one can imagine, establishing this causal relationship is not easy because women who are OC users are less likely to use barrier methods such as condoms which, in turn, may put them at an increased risk for HPV.

It is also relevant to point out the effects of hormones on the transformation zone. It is thought that perhaps the influence of the hormone estrogen, present in birth control pills, maintains the transformation zone on the exocervix for a longer period of time; doing so facilitates the direct exposure of the cervix to HPV and other STIs. In addition, the pill, being a steroid derivative, may weaken the immune system in the long run and increase the persistence of HPV infections.

> ☞ **The overall risk of cervical cancer from oral contraceptives is small.**

In addition, there is some evidence to suggest that the small increase in risk of cervical cancer due to OCs may drop after one stops taking them. More research is required, however, to confirm these findings (Smith et al. 2003). The important things to remember are to follow safe sexual practices and obtain regular gynecological exams from your health-care professional.

Genetics

Genetic makeup is one risk factor that cannot be changed. Though research is still underway, it seems that genetics can increase the susceptibility of getting cervical cancer. According to the American Cancer

Society, a woman's chances of getting cervical cancer are increased two to threefold if her mother or sister has had the disease. Similarly, genetics may also play a role in making some women less able to stave off HPV infections. And while it is important to know the risk factors that can be changed, it is even *more* important to know the risk factors that cannot be changed, so that one can take extra precautions to minimize the risk.

Male Cofactors

Men who have not been circumcised have a higher rate of HPV infections and are more likely to transmit them to their sexual partners. HPV likes to reside in the warm, moist area under the foreskin that covers the tip of the penis. Studies have shown that circumcision can reduce the rates of HPV transmission. Similarly, condoms have been shown to reduce the rate of HPV transmission by 70 percent. Male cofactors are discussed in greater detail in Chapter 7.

Ethnic Minorities

Despite widespread screening programs in the United States, there are still nearly 4,000 women every year who die of cervical cancer. Research shows that African American women are at a 60 percent higher risk for developing the invasive disease and have about twice the risk of dying from cervical cancer than their Caucasian counterparts in the United States (Ries et al. 2006). Hispanic and American Indian women and Asian immigrants also have higher than average death rates from cervical cancer. Financial restraints, poor access to health care, lack of insurance, inadequate public education about HPV and other STIs, and increased substance abuse are some of the main reasons for the heightened prevalence in poor-resource communities. Additional barriers include language problems, cultural and social differences, and poor compliance, all of which account for the increased risk of cervical cancer in this underprivileged population.

In developing countries, 80 percent of all cases of cervical cancers and 85 percent of the deaths from cervical cancer occur in women due to poor awareness and lack of cervical screening programs such as the Pap test (a test that checks for abnormal changes in the cells of the cervix). Not having access to regular screening allows cervical cancer to go undetected until its later stages and increases the death rates from it.

Gays, Lesbians, and Bisexuals

Like most ethnic minorities, the lesbian, gay, bisexual, transgender, and queer (LGBTQ) communities often face social, cultural, and financial barriers when trying to access health care. Many withhold their sexual orientation due to fear of discrimination. It has been observed that there is also a higher incidence of stress, smoking, and substance abuse in this population, which leads to high-risk behaviors such as multiple partners, unprotected sex, and higher incidence of HPV (ACS). Transgender care is not normally taught in schools in the United States, and health-care providers are not well equipped to deal with LGBTQ issues. This results in a general distrust within this population toward the health-care community to be well versed in their needs. In addition, poor access to medical insurance compared to heterosexual couples (since many insurance companies and employers do not provide domestic partnership benefits) also makes it difficult for members of the LGBTQ community to afford good health care. In other words, the societal effects of being gay play a major role in the prevalence of HPV-related diseases in this community.

Many people believe that cervical cancer rates would be low among lesbians. However, according to the National Institutes of Health (NIH), cervical cancer rates may actually be higher in lesbian women for several reasons. As genital HPV is spread through skin-to-skin contact or tiny breaks in the skin, transmission can occur between female-to-female partner sexual activity. Because lesbians believe that they will not get cervical cancer unless they have sex with men, they are more likely to engage in unprotected sexual acts that cause such skin-to-skin contact. It is also possible that they could have been in heterosexual relationships in the past and may continue to do so at irregular intervals.

Lesbians also may be more likely to avoid getting their Pap tests due to past negative experiences. The majority of health-care providers assume female patients to be heterosexual and only inquire about the number of male partners they have been with and assume that they are taking birth control pills.

An overview of HPV risk factors is shown in Table 3.2.

Table 3.2 HPV Risk Factors Overview

Risk factors that *fire* HPV infections	Risk factors that *add fuel to the fire*
Sexual contact at an early age	HPV infections
History of having multiple sexual partners	A weakened immune system; factors include stress, medications, HIV, poor diet, other STIs, etc.
Having sexual relationship with a partner who has had multiple partners	Tobacco smoking
Sexual contact with a partner who is infected	Birth control pills
Frequency of sexual intercourse	Being an ethnic minority, sexual minority (such as gay, lesbian and bisexual), and woman in the developing world

TESTING

Now that we have discussed the primary risk factors for HPV infections and cervical cancer, the next step is to discuss how you can get tested for HPV. It is important to note that unlike HIV, there is no blood test for HPV because the virus is "silent" and mostly undetectable. It does not produce any ripples in the blood count or the immune system. In fact, the only way in which the immune system can recognize the presence of HPV is when it releases proteins into the blood during an active infection. But when the virus lies dormant in the basal cells (the bottommost layer of the epithelium), it keeps itself relatively invisible and escapes detection by releasing no or very minimal proteins.

Because a more conventional blood test does not exist for the detection of HPV, scientists have had to devise different tests and other ways to detect HPV. These tests fall under two main categories—the indirect method (the Pap test) and the direct method, which involves HPV genetic testing that directly detects HPV DNA in the cervical cells.

The Indirect Method—Pap Test (Also Called Pap Smear)

The Pap test (named after Dr. George N. Papanicolaou, who developed this test) is perhaps the most effective cancer screening method ever devised in the history of preventive medicine. Even today, it remains the gold standard for early detection of cervical cancer. In the United States, the Pap test has dramatically reduced the disease burden and deaths related to cervical cancer by 75 percent in the past 50 years (Ries et al. 2006). In other words, the Pap test has decreased the incidence of cervical cancer from 30–40 per 100,000 women to 8 per 100,000. According to the American Cancer Society, cervical cancer was once the leading cause of cancer death in women. But now, it is not even among the top ten in the list of cancer deaths in the United States. In addition, studies have shown that the introduction of Pap tests to populations that have never been screened before reduces the risk of cervical cancer rates by 60–90 percent within three years of implementation (IARC 2005).

The goal of the Pap test is to sample the highly susceptible transformation zone (TZ), the area where physiologic transformation from columnar (endocervical) epithelium to squamous (ectocervical) epithelium takes place and where cancerous changes occur. As discussed earlier, the TZ changes its location from the ectocervix to the endocervix

> ☞ **The Pap test is the gold standard for detecting abnormal cell changes in the cervix that may be caused by HPV.**

with increasing age. Hence, scrapings for the Pap test are taken from both the ectocervix and the endocervix. A Pap test does not look for HPV directly, but instead looks for changes in the cervical cells induced by HPV infections. Results are reported as either the cells being normal in appearance, or having varying degrees of abnormalities; these abnormalities are also called dysplasias or intraepithelial lesions. (This will be discussed in greater detail in Chapter 4.)

So, How Is a Pap Test Done?

During a Pap test, you are asked to lie down on the exam table for a pelvic exam. A steel or a plastic speculum, a duck-beak-like instrument, is carefully introduced into the vagina so that the cervix can be brought into view. A wooden spatula or a brush that looks like a long mascara wand is then introduced into the os, the opening of the cervix (see Figure 2.2), and twirled to get a scraping of the tissue. The sample is then either spread on a glass slide and preserved with a fixative (the conventional method), or the brush is rinsed in a small container of fixative (the liquid-based method, also called the Thin Prep) and transported to the lab to undergo testing.

Who Should Get a Pap Test?

You should have your first Pap test at age 21 or three years after sexual debut, whichever comes first, as per the guidelines of the American Cancer Society (see Table 3.3).

Table 3.3 Guidelines for Pap Tests in the United States

Age	Frequency
Below 21	Pap test is recommended if a woman has already been sexually active for 3 years or more.
21–29	· Once a year if conventional Pap test is used. · Once every other year if liquid-based Pap test is used.
30–69	· Once every 2 to 3 years if previous three Pap tests have been normal. · Once every 3 years if previous Pap and HPV DNA tests are negative. · Once yearly if a woman is HIV positive, has been exposed to DES in the mother's womb, or is taking a medication that can weaken the body's immune system, such as a steroid.
70 and older	· Discontinue Pap tests if 3 consecutive Pap smears in the past 10 years have been normal. · Continue Pap tests if medical history or sexual history warrants follow-up. Follow your health-care provider's recommendations.

Source: Based on information from the American Cancer Society.

Pap Tests in Special Circumstances

Regardless of age, if you have certain risk factors, your doctor may suggest an annual Pap test. Some of the important risk factors include multiple sexual partners at the present time, HIV infection, or a weakened immune system due to factors such as an organ transplant, chemotherapy (medication for treatment of cancer), or chronic use of steroid medications.

Pap Tests after Hysterectomy

Under normal circumstances, women who have had a total hysterectomy (removal of uterus and cervix) for any benign condition can stop having Pap tests. The exception to this case would be when the patient underwent the procedure as a part of the treatment for cervical cancer. If the hysterectomy was for a precancerous or cancerous condition, the vaginal canal should still be checked for abnormal changes. Also, women who have had their cervix left behind, as in partial or subtotal hysterectomy (where the uterus is surgically removed but the cervix is left in place), should continue to follow the guidelines above.

Pap Tests in Older Women

Unfortunately, many people share the myth that once a woman has passed her reproductive age, she does not require a Pap test. Data from a National Health Interview Survey in 1992 showed that one-half of all women aged 60 and older had not had a Pap test in the three years prior. Continuation of such a trend could be devastating as one in four cases of cervical cancer, and 41 percent of cervical cancer deaths occur in women 65 and older; this is because HPV can lie dormant and resurface several years later to cause cervical cancer. The American Cancer Society recommends Pap smears for women until 70 years of age.

Anal Pap Tests

Anal Pap tests are similar to cervical Pap tests. Just as cervical Pap tests are performed in women having vaginal intercourse, anal Pap tests can be performed in men and women having anal intercourse in order to detect abnormal changes in the anal canal that may lead to anal cancer. There are many similarities between the cell lining of the anal canal and the cervix. For that reason the Pap test lends itself equally well to anal screening. The liquid-based method is usually used for anal Pap tests.

Anal Pap tests, though not routine, are being used in several research studies and in some private clinics among high-risk individuals such as gay men, HIV-positive men and women, commercial sex workers, and women who have had anal intercourse with multiple sex partners. Nearly 90 percent of anal cancers are caused by HPV.

There are no specific guidelines for anal Pap tests as there is poor awareness among the general public and health-care providers alike about anal cancers and their early detection. Some experts, however, recommend performing anal Pap tests on a yearly basis on HIV-positive men and to proceed with biopsy for any positive results. In non–HIV-positive men who participate in receptive anal sex, the general recommendations are to obtain a baseline anal Pap test at age 40 and follow up every two to three years. Anal cancer, like cervical cancer, is a very slow-growing disease that typically appears in people over the age of 50, and most often in people over the age of 65.

Accuracy: How Reliable Are Pap Tests?

As mentioned earlier, the Pap test is one of the best cancer screening tests ever devised; it has proven to be extremely effective in detecting the precursors of cervical cancer. However, as effective a test as it may be, the Pap test is not perfect. In order to better appreciate this, we have to first understand the terms "sensitivity" and "specificity."

All patients undergoing testing for any disease or condition fall into two broad categories—those who have the disease or condition, and those who do not. The term commonly used when a patient who *has* the disease or condition and *tests positive* is a "true positive." Similarly, the term used when a patient who is *free* of the disease or condition and *tests negative* is "true negative." Keeping this in mind, sensitivity and specificity—the terms most widely used in statistics to describe the validity of any diagnostic test—can be explained as follows:

- Sensitivity is the probability of detecting a "true positive" among patients who have the disease, and
- Specificity is the probability of detecting a "true negative" among patients free of the disease.

A Pap test done once has a sensitivity of only 50–80 percent. This means it will only pick up a true positive 50–80 percent of the time when done once on a given patient. This may not sound impressive, as it may miss many true positives, but if done at regular intervals over time, its cumulative sensitivity will give us ample opportunity to diagnose and treat abnormal Pap smears. Because HPV generally takes years, if not decades, to progress from an abnormal precancerous lesion to cervical cancer, Pap tests done at regular intervals will be able to detect abnormal cervical changes in the early and treatable stages. Therefore, the effectiveness of a Pap test lies in its *repetition.* According to the American College of Pathology, four out of five women who die of cervical cancer did not have a Pap smear in the five years preceding their deaths.

One of the pitfalls of a Pap test is that it can be misread. A test result can be incorrectly read as normal, even though cancer or precancerous cells are present. Such a test result is called a "false negative." Inadequate sampling and improper slide preparation may be responsible for 90–95 percent of all false negatives. False negatives can fail to recognize or correctly classify abnormal cells, and, as such, every precaution must be taken to eliminate or minimize them.

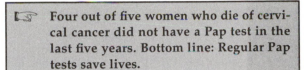

Four out of five women who die of cervical cancer did not have a Pap test in the last five years. Bottom line: Regular Pap tests save lives.

On the flip side, a test result can be incorrectly read as abnormal, even though there are no cancerous or precancerous cells present on the smear. Such a test result is called a "false positive." False positives incorrectly indicate that cancer or precancerous lesions are present in a normal cell sample. Because this can naturally lead to a great deal of anxiety and confusion for the patient, every precaution should be taken to avoid this, too.

On the whole, a Pap test, in spite of its deficiencies, is considered to be an excellent screening test. It is relatively inexpensive, easy to administer, and, if done at predetermined intervals, detects a potentially serious disease in its early stages for which effective treatment is available. This results in a significant reduction in the number of complications and deaths resulting from the disease.

The Direct Method—HPV DNA Testing: Is It the Wave of the Future?

There is now an increasingly growing interest worldwide in the potential use for HPV DNA testing in cervical cancer prevention programs. Unlike Pap tests, which screen for abnormal cell changes of the cervix, HPV DNA tests detect the genetic material of the virus and can tell if a woman has high-risk HPV types. The HPV DNA test has a specificity and sensitivity of greater than 94 percent, which is impressive (Mayrand et al. 2007). But the HPV DNA test is not for every woman. Then, who should get it?

Who Should Get the HPV DNA Test? Age Matters

There are two reasons for which the HPV DNA test is administered. One is as a primary screening along with a Pap smear in women 30 and older. This is also known as a DNA Pap test. The second is a triage test when women over the age of 20 years have an abnormal and inconclusive Pap smear result. The test is done to confirm if the abnormality in the cervical cells is due to the high-risk HPV or other reasons such as a bacterial or yeast infection.

Though the HPV DNA test sounds like the perfect test that should be applied to women of all ages, it too is not without limitations. One major obstacle to administering this test is its high cost. The HPV test can cost anywhere between $50 and $100 compared with as little as $20 for a Pap test. More significantly, many sexually active women will be infected with HPV at some point in their lives. Therefore, the need to balance the cost of testing every woman versus the resulting benefits has to be weighed. Also, its usefulness in women less than 30 years old is limited, because 90 percent of HPV infections in this age group clear on their own within 2 years. Therefore, performing tests for an infection that is going to resolve itself in the majority of cases would be not only an unnecessary emotional burden on the patient, as she would be subjected to numerous follow-up tests and procedures, but also a waste of precious time, resources, and money.

HPV DNA testing as a primary screening test makes practical sense in women over 30 years of age. Cervical cancer is a slow-growing cancer that peaks between the ages of 35 and 50. Most infections that do not resolve by themselves occur after age 30. Therefore, testing for persistence in this age group would be beneficial in order to find out which women may be at a greater risk for cervical cancer. A study showed that in women over age 30 the sensitivity of the Pap test and the HPV DNA test combined was 100 percent and the specificity was 92.5 percent (Mayrand et al. 2007). Clinical trials have also shown that the addition of a HPV DNA test to the Pap test to screen women in their thirties and older for cervical cancers reduces the incidence of more severe forms of abnormal Pap smears detected in subsequent screening exams. This is why the American Cancer Society recommends HPV DNA testing in all women after the age of 30, in addition to a Pap test. So, if a woman after 30 has a normal Pap smear but is HPV DNA positive, her health-care provider may choose to observe her more closely and perform a Pap test more often than otherwise indicated to look for early cervical changes. It is worth mentioning again that doctors can only treat the changes to cells that HPV may cause, but they cannot treat the virus.

Techniques for Detecting HPV—How Is It Done?

HPV cannot be reliably cultured in a laboratory setting, nor can it be detected in the blood. Therefore, molecular techniques are employed to recognize the HPV DNA protein in cervical cell samples.

There is only one commercially available HPV DNA test, Digene Corporation's Hybrid Capture 2 (HC2) assay that is currently licensed by the FDA for clinical use. This test was approved in the United States in 1999. It detects 13 high-risk HPV types (16, 18, 31, 33, 35, 39, 45, 51, 52, 56, 58, 59, and 68) and is standardized and highly reproducible. The test checks for all these high-risk HPV strains as a group and does not have the capability to detect each individual type. Therefore, in order to accomplish this, two newer products are seeking FDA approval in the near future. One will be an alternative to the current HPV DNA testing option and will screen for 14 of the high-risk HPV infections. This test will detect the proteins that are released when these infections progress toward cervical cancer. The other new test will determine if a patient is infected with HPV type 16 or 18, the two most carcinogenic types. These tests will generate tremendous interest in light of the recent FDA approval of the HPV vaccine.

As a patient, you will not know the difference between the conduct of the Pap test and the test for HPV DNA. Either a separate brush will be used to collect the cervical smear, or in the case of a Thin Prep, the test can be performed from the same specimen.

How Is the Test Interpreted?

Your HPV Pap test result will return as either normal (high-risk HPV is not present) or abnormal, meaning one or more high-risk types of HPV are present. An abnormal result indicates that you may be at increased risk of having precancerous cervical changes and further testing may be required. Your DNA Pap test will either come back HPV negative or positive. Done together, the two tests yield four possible results:

Negative HPV, Normal Pap Test
This result is the best outcome for all. If you have negative HPV testing and a normal Pap smear test (remember, HPV DNA testing is done along with a Pap smear as a routine only in those over the age of 30 years), there is a 99 percent chance that you are free of any HPV. An added benefit to this is that the patient can undergo follow-up testing on a less frequent basis as determined by the physician.

Negative HPV, Abnormal Pap Test
If you have an abnormal Pap smear and a negative HPV, then your cervical abnormality is most likely due to low-risk HPV or non-HPV infections. It could also be that the Pap smear could have been a false positive and that you really did not have the abnormal cells. Regardless, when you have an abnormal Pap smear, your health-care professional might recommend you to come sooner than the standard protocol, to obtain a follow-up Pap smear until you test negative.

As we discussed earlier, in women less than 30 years of age, DNA testing is not routinely done because over 90 percent of the infections resolve spontaneously. In our office, we have the lab do the DNA testing in women aged 20 and older only if the Pap smear result is abnormal and inconclusive due to a condition called ASCUS (atypical squamous cells of unknown significance), which we will discuss in detail in the next chapter. This information can be useful to your clinician to better understand and document the reason for the inconclusive Pap.

Positive HPV, Normal Pap Test

A positive HPV test means that you have HPV on your cervix. It indicates that you are infected with one or more high-risk HPV types that could put you at an increased risk of developing cell changes, which, in turn, could lead to cervical cancer over time. This *does not* mean that you have or will get cervical cancer. Even if the Pap is normal, your health-care provider might decide to follow up by testing you more frequently.

Positive HPV, Abnormal Pap Test

This is the most undesirable outcome, as both tests show abnormalities. If you have a positive HPV test and an abnormal Pap smear, you may be asked to undergo a procedure called a "colposcopy" as the next step. Colposcopy is a procedure in which the cervix is examined using a bright light and magnification. Often a biopsy (a small pea-sized piece of tissue) of the infected area is taken and sent to a pathology lab for examination and further appropriate management. See Table 3.4 for the different possible results when both the Pap test and an HPV DNA test are administered.

The HPV DNA test is much more sensitive than the Pap test, which is now a yearly ritual for many women. Pap tests have been the core of cervical cancer prevention for over the past 50 years. However, with the emerging interest in the role of HPV DNA testing as the primary screening test in women over 30 years of age, the Pap test may start to fade in importance in the coming years if the adoption of the HPV DNA test becomes the test of choice in women over the age of 30. The HPV DNA test could monitor the risk and provide the much-needed early warning

Table 3.4 HPV DNA Pap Test Results

Test results	Pap test normal	Pap test abnormal
HPV negative	Follow routine cancer screening protocol.	Abnormal Pap due to non-high-risk HPV or non-HPV types. Low risk of cancer. Follow up according to protocol or your health-care provider's recommendations.
HPV positive	HPV picked up before cellular changes. Does not mean you will get cervical cancer. Your health-care provider may choose to see you sooner for a repeat Pap test.	You may require further testing and procedures as determined by your health-care provider.

that could eventually reduce the mortality rates from cervical cancer and relieve the pervasive misery that the disease causes worldwide.

HPV Testing in Men
Even though men are 50 percent of the "problem" in the spread of HPV, there are no HPV tests currently approved in males. As is the case with cervical Pap smears in women, some doctors are screening high-risk men with anal Pap smears on a case-by-case basis. Testing in men is described in greater detail in Chapter 7.

KEY FACTS

- HPV infections are necessary but not sufficient to cause cervical cancer or other HPV-related diseases on their own.
- Persistence of HPV infections is a major factor in the development of cancer precursors.
- Smoking prolongs HPV infections in both men and women, which in turn can lead to HPV-related cancer.
- The risk of cervical cancer from the pill is small.
- The Pap test is still the gold standard for early detection of cervical cancer.
- HPV DNA testing could become the primary screening test in women over 30 in the future.
- Having a robust immune system through a healthy lifestyle is the key to minimizing risk from HPV infections.

4

CANCER, WARTS, AND HPV: FROM HEAD AND NECK LESIONS TO CERVICAL, PENILE, AND ANAL DISEASES

Myth: HPV infections only cause cervical cancers.

Fact: HPV infections can cause a variety of diseases, ranging from warts to cancers in both in men and women.

The medical costs associated with treating HPV-related diseases in the United States are second only to the costs created by HIV/AIDS. Yet, research shows that the knowledge of HPV among the public is poor (Tirol et al. 2007). Myths and misconceptions are widespread even among those who have heard of HPV. For example, few women know the links between genital HPV infections, abnormal Pap smears, and cervical cancer. Even fewer people are aware of the broad spectrum of HPV-related diseases that ranges from relatively harmless, albeit unsightly, genital warts to the more perilous cervical, vulval, vaginal, oral, and anal cancers. And sadly, the majority of the public is completely oblivious to the numerous HPV diseases that can be manifested in men, including genital warts and oral, anal, and penile cancers.

HPV infections are not only a health hazard for the individual but also an economic burden to society. Women carry the brunt of the burden, as cervical cancer is the most serious consequence of HPV infection and carries the greatest threat to life. Approximately over $4 billion is spent annually in the diagnosis and treatment of HPV infections and their associated cervical diseases in the United States alone (Insinga et al. 2004). Out of this, nearly $2 billion is spent on routine cervical screening, another $2 billion on follow-up of abnormal Pap smears, and $350 million on invasive cervical cancer procedures.

In addition to this, approximately another $200 million is spent on treating genital warts in both men and women (Chesson et al. 2004). Of the total estimated monies spent on HPV-related cervical disease, approximately 90 percent is spent on strategies for the prevention of cervical cancer: routines like Pap smears and the follow-up and treatment of abnormal Pap smears. The other 10 percent is spent on the treatment of cervical cancer. Most of the expenditures on HPV infections are incurred by the 15–24 age group, as these are the years when HPV infections peak. From an economic standpoint, one can see that the burden of cervical cancer in a developed country such as the United States is small; this is entirely due to an established and successful cervical screening program—the Pap test, which has reduced the rates of cervical cancer by 75 percent in the past 50 years.

In addition to women, men can also manifest the benign and malignant clinical presentations of HPV infections, thus rendering the disease a significant consequence for both genders. In addition to the more obvious costs, HPV infections are also responsible for many of the psychological aspects associated with sexually transmitted diseases—emotional, social, and sexual trauma for which a direct dollar value cannot be ascertained.

This chapter has been designed to provide a deeper understanding of some of the most common and serious of HPV disease manifestations: from the most common and benign (genital warts) to the most life threatening (cervical cancer). Because conditions such as Recurrent Respiratory Papillomas (RRPs), cancers of the mouth and throat, and of course, penile cancers due to HPV are more common in men than women, they are discussed in Chapter 7 (HPV Vaccines for Males).

HPV-HIV LINK

Most HPV infections progress to dysplasias and cancer depending on the integrity of the person's immune system. As a weakened immune system is the hallmark of HIV/AIDS, those inflicted with this disease also have a higher chance of a potential HPV infection progressing to cancer. This is true in both women and men. For example, in HIV-positive women, the incidence of anal cancer is about seven times higher than that of HIV-negative women, and in HIV-positive men, the incidence of anal cancer is almost 37 times higher than that of HIV-negative men. Genital warts in HIV/AIDS patients can also spread aggressively and undergo cancerous transformations.

HPV-RELATED DISEASES

A brief summary of the pertinent HPV-associated conditions, along with their incidence, is provided in Table 4.1.

Table 4.1 Approximate Numbers of HPV-associated Conditions in Males and Females in the United States per Year

HPV-associated conditions	Estimated cases/year
Genital warts	1 million
Cervical dysplasia (mild)	1–1.4 million
Cervical dysplasia (moderate to severe)	330,000
Recurrent respiratory papillomas	6,000
Cervical cancer	11,000
Anal cancer	4,700
Vulvar cancer	3,500
Vaginal cancer	2,200
Penile cancer	1,000
Mouth and throat cancer	11,000
Total	**2.3–2.8 million**

Source: Based on information from the American Cancer Society.

Genital Warts

Genital warts (also called condyloma acuminata or venereal warts) are the most commonly recognized and frustrating manifestation of HPV infections. Any person who is sexually active can get genital warts. However, not all persons infected with HPV 6 or 11 acquire genital warts. Warts can appear in various forms on different sites of the body. Some HPV types, such as types 1, 2, and 4, prefer to reside on the skin of the hands and feet, while types 6, 11, 16, and 18 like to reside in the genital area. Approximately 1 percent of sexually active people in the United States have genital warts (Koutsky 1997). Nearly 1 million new cases of genital warts occur each year in the United States. All genital warts are caused by HPV, with 90 percent of them being caused by HPV types 6 and 11 (Greer et al. 1995).

Genital warts are spread by sexual activity, and they carry a much more pernicious threat than warts on the hands or feet. Genital warts can also be spread by skin-to-skin contact during vaginal, anal, or (rarely) oral sex with someone who is infected. In addition, they are very contagious and recurrent. About two-thirds of people who have had sexual contact with a partner with genital warts will develop them between six weeks to nine months after contact.

Genital warts may be raised or flat, small or large, and can occur alone or in clusters. They are soft to touch and usually painless. They can occur in women on the vulva and inside and surrounding the vagina and anus. In men, genital warts can appear on the scrotum or penis. In addition, genital warts can also occur in the pubic area and on the upper inner sides of thighs. Genital warts not only are unsightly, but they can also cause discomfort such as itching and bleeding. In the majority of cases, they are benign and do not turn into cancer, although there is one genetic condition called epidermodysplasia verruciformis (luckily, one does not have to pronounce this condition very often as it a rare occurrence) where malignant changes take place. This condition provided one of the initial clues to scientists that HPV might cause cancer. It appears early in life with generalized warts on the body, and it undergoes life-threatening cancerous transformation.

Even though genital warts, unlike epidermodysplasia verruciformis, are not life threatening, they are highly contagious and can transmit freely. They are also associated with other health problems; their presence can signify exposure to other types of HPV that include the cancer-causing types. The open sores that may result from scratching or other trauma to genital warts can also increase the risk for the HIV virus to gain access more freely in those exposed to it. In addition, warts can cause psychological symptoms such as depression, stress, poor self-esteem, and anxiety.

Treatment

Because there is no cure for HPV, several treatment options have been tried for genital warts; from folk remedies such as rubbing a dusty dry toad on warts to laser surgery. Warts can resolve spontaneously, recur, or be resistant to treatment. Whatever the case may be, there is no evidence to show that removal of warts will reduce transmission, as the infectious material could also be contained in the surrounding tissue. Some specialists believe that removal of warts will nevertheless reduce the viral load at that site. Regardless of whether removal of warts helps or not, most people understandably like to get rid of their warts for physical, psychological, and social reasons.

Because warts have no known cure, the effectiveness of any treatment depends on several critical determining factors: the patient's age, host immunity, compliance with treatment, wart location and size, number of warts, treatment method used, and the clinical experience of the professional administering the treatment. It should also be noted that none of the treatments has yet proven to be 100 percent effective. Both surgical and nonsurgical methods are used and repeated treatments may be required. The following are the most frequently use methods:

Surgical methods

- Simple excision—cutting with a scalpel.
- Electrocautery—burning the warts with an electric current.
- Cryosurgery—freezing the warts with liquid nitrogen.

- Laser therapy—using an intense light to remove warts (reserved for large and extensive warts that are hard to remove or have not responded to other treatments).

Nonsurgical methods

- Imiquimod cream (Aldara®)—a topical treatment that stimulates the body's immune system to destroy warts. It is a self-applied treatment for external genital warts that is safe, effective, and easy to use. Recently, an ointment with green tea extract has also been approved for this purpose.
- Podofilox cream or gel (Condylox®)—also a self-applied treatment that destroys warts by preventing their cells from dividing.
- 20% Podophyllin solution—Podophyllin, a chemical compound that must be applied by a doctor or nurse, is an older treatment and is not as widely used today.
- Bichloroacetic acid (BCA)—a solution applied at the doctor's office that destroys genital warts by coagulating the protein in the infected cells.
- Trichloroacetic acid (TCA)—works similarly to BCA by destroying the protein in the wart cells.
- Interferon injections—a substance that is injected into warts. It acts by stimulating the body's immune system to fight off the HPV. It is rarely used because of its high cost and extensive side effects Also, less expensive alternatives work just as well.
- Bleomycin injections—an anticancer medication that is used to stop the growth of nongenital warts if other topical treatments do not help.

Although these treatments will generally get rid of the warts, it is very important to note that none can get rid of the virus. In other words, getting rid of warts does not automatically mean that one is free from the possibility of transmitting the virus asymptomatically. In addition, recurrences of warts are common regardless of whether they clear spontaneously or after treatment (Chuang et al. 1984). The cost of a successful treatment course can be several hundred dollars.

One final concern about genital warts involves their possible transmission from pregnant women to their children. Genital warts can grow bigger during pregnancy as a result of the change in hormonal balance, but seldom do they obstruct the vaginal passage for delivery. Almost all children delivered vaginally to women with genital warts are born healthy, but a small number develop warts in their respiratory tract (airway passages) as a result of passing through an infected birth canal. Despite this, Cesarean section (C-section) births are not automatically recommended for women with HPV. Children of infected mothers delivered by C-section have also developed warts, and hence, the pros and cons of each individual case are best left to the physician and the patient.

In addition to warts, HPV can cause dysplasias and cancer in other parts of the genital areas. They are as follows:

HPV-Related Vaginal Dysplasias and Cancers

The vagina is the gateway to the female reproductive system. As it is an organ that is exposed to the outside environment, it is subject to various kinds of trauma by objects such as tampons during menstrual cycles, the penis during sexual intercourse, and the baby during childbirth, to name a few. Irritation and abrasions to the vaginal lining by any of these objects facilitate the HPV's ability to gain access into the basal cell layer. Like the cervix, the vaginal lining is made up of two main cell types—the squamous epithelial cells, and the glandular cells—both of which can undergo abnormal transformation, or dysplasia, that may progress to cancer. (As a reference, note that the vagina is the birth canal, different from the cervix, which is the lower part of the uterus. Refer to Figure 2.2.)

Vaginal cancer is a rare disease. According to National Cancer Institute estimates, there were about 2,140 new cases of vaginal cancer and 790 deaths in the United States in 2007. Nearly 85 percent of vaginal cancers are squamous cell carcinomas that start in the thin, flat cells that line the vagina. Another 10–15 percent are adenocarcinomas, a cancer that begins in glandular cells of the vaginal lining. Approximately 50 percent of vaginal dysplasias and cancers are HPV related, with HPV 16 being the most common type (Daling et al. 2002). The cause for the other 50 percent is mostly unknown.

Most squamous cell carcinomas and vaginal adenocarcinomas develop in women after the age of 50. However, one special type of adenocarcinoma of the vagina, called "clear cell" adenocarcinoma, develops in women who were exposed to the drug DES while they were in their mother's womb. As discussed earlier, DES was a drug used by women in the 1940s to the 1970s to prevent miscarriages. It was banned in the United States in 1971. DES-related adenocarcinomas are, however, extremely rare.

Most vaginal dysplasias (also called vaginal intraepithelial neoplasias or VAIN) and early vaginal cancer do not present with any symptoms. Sometimes, one may notice a vaginal lump or bleeding that is not a menstrual period.

A Pap test is the best defense against vaginal cancer, because cells obtained from the cervix are often mixed with vaginal cells. Any abnormal vaginal cells present can thus be detected for early cancer. Vaginal cancer can be cured in its early stages with cure rates as high as 96 percent (ACS).

Treatment

There are several methods to treat vaginal and other HPV-related cancers. Following is a glossary of terms of procedures that are employed in treating cancers:

Surgery

Surgery involves removal of the cancerous area and its surrounding tissue. Depending on the extent of the cancer, the surgery could be either minimal or very invasive.

Radiation Therapy

Radiation therapy is the use of high-energy rays to shrink cancer cells. Radiation therapy is either external or internal. In external radiation, a large machine beams radiation onto the body where the cancer is located. In internal radiation therapy, devices filled with radioactive material are placed in an area close to the cancer. Radiation therapy can be used alone or in combination with surgery and chemotherapy.

Chemotherapy

Chemotherapy is the use of potent anticancer medications to destroy the cancer cells. These medications, administered orally or intravenously, enter the body's bloodstream and shrink the tumor cells. Chemotherapeutic drugs act synergistically with radiation to treat cancer.

Radical Hysterectomy

A radial hysterectomy is the removal of the whole uterus including the cervix, part of the vagina, and neighboring lymph nodes. This is the standard treatment in earlier stages of invasive cervical cancer.

Radical Trachelectomy

Radical trachelectomy is a procedure that preserves fertility in young women who have early stages of cervical cancer. This procedure involves removing the cervix and the lower part of the uterus. The rest of the uterus is left behind in order to carry the pregnancy. Lymph nodes in the pelvis are also removed during this procedure to determine whether the cancer has spread.

HPV-Related Vulvar Dysplasias and Cancers

Cancer of the vulva (the vulva is the external female genital organ that includes the vaginal lips and the clitoris) is rare and slow growing. According to National Cancer Institute estimates, there were 3,490 new cases of vulvar cancers and 880 deaths from it in the United States in 2007. Nevertheless, vulvar cancers are important gynecological cancers because of the role they play in a woman's sexuality.

Ninety percent of vulvar cancers stem from the squamous cells. About 50 percent are related to HPV, and most others stem from a chronic skin condition of the vulva. However, due to the rising rates of HPV infections in the past two to three decades, there has also been a rise in the rates of vulvar cancers in women under the age of 40. Nearly 15 percent of vulvar cancers are currently seen in this age group.

Most of the vulvar cancers cause no symptoms. But, in those cases that do, discolorations, lumps, or bleeding can be easily recognized by the patient. Vulvar dysplasias and cancers can be caused by two separate diseases. The first type develops as a result of HPV infections, and the second type, which afflicts older women, usually develops from a chronic skin condition called Lichen sclerosis. This condition causes persistent itching and inflammation of the skin of the vulva. These changes are usually detected by women and reported to their health-care professionals (Judson et al. 2006).

Treatment

Not all vulvar dysplasias (also called vulvar intraepithelial neoplasia or VIN) progress to cancer, but, if cancer is detected, treatment outcomes remain good. Depending on the specific type of vulvar cancer and how advanced it is, treatment options may include surgery, radiation, and chemotherapy. Recent trends in surgery have taken a more conservative approach toward salvaging the vulvar tissue in order to decrease the psychological and the social impact of the disease.

HPV-Related Anal Diseases

"Anal sex" is taboo and is highly stigmatized in many societies including the United States, probably because anal intercourse is mostly associated with homosexuality. However, it is a form of sexual expression that has been practiced not only by homosexuals but also by bisexuals and heterosexuals for centuries. One has to look at premodern cultural literature and art to understand that anal sex was prevalent in olden times, and it continues to be the case in modern times as well. According to CDC estimates in 2005, nearly 20–40 percent of heterosexual couples have engaged in anal sex at least once, and for 10 percent of heterosexual couples it is a part of their regular sexual repertoire. Therefore, in absolute numbers, anal cancers are, surprisingly, more common in women than in men, as there are more women having receptive anal sex than men. The incidence of anal cancer continues to rise in women every year as women's attitudes toward anal sex change and more and more women engage in anal intercourse.

According to estimates from the American Cancer Society in 2007, about 4,650 new cases of anal cancer were diagnosed in the United States that year, out of which nearly 2,750 occurred in women and 1,900 occurred in men. An estimated 430 women and 260 men died from it, resulting in a total of 690 deaths in 2007. Anal cancer is more common among African Americans and in people over the age of 50.

HPV-related anal lesions are of special significance among men having sex with men (MSM)—gay and bisexual men. In this chapter, we will briefly review HPV-related anal diseases and anal cancer in the general population. Anal cancer in gay and bisexual men is discussed in detail in Chapter 7.

Anal sex carries two principle risks: infections, due to the inherent nature of organisms found in the anal canal, and damage to its mucous membrane because of decreased natural lubrication at the site, making it more vulnerable to microorganisms including HPV.

Anatomically, the mucus lining of the anus has a lot in common with the cervical lining. It has a transformation zone (TZ), where the columnar cells of the rectum meet the squamous cells of the anus about 2–4 centimeters inside the anal canal. As in the case of the cervix, HPV likes to infect the anal transformation zone. HPV can cause warts, dysplasias, and cancer in the perianal area and the anal canal. Ninety percent of anal cancers are caused by HPV 16 and 18, with HPV 16 causing the majority of them. Most anal warts are caused by HPV 6 and 11.

Many people have no symptoms with anal dysplasia or with early stages of anal cancer. When symptoms do occur, a person may present with anal itching or a sore or bump in the anal area. Symptoms such as discharge, bleeding, pain or pressure around the anus may also occur.

Diagnosis of anal diseases can be established in several ways, including:

- Rectal exam—a manual exam by the clinician to look for any abnormal bumps.
- Anal Pap smears—a test to look for abnormal cells from the TZ under a microscope. However, this is not standard practice. Some doctors recommend anal Pap smears for HIV-positve men and women, women who are commercial sex workers, women with genital warts (as they are more prone to be infected with other types of HPV), or women with vaginal, vulvar, or cervical dysplasias or cancer.
- Anoscopy—a scope is inserted into the anal canal to look at the area directly.
- Biopsy—surgically removing a piece of the tissue for clinical testing.

Treatment

Treatments for anal cancers include surgery, radiation, and chemotherapy. Treatment for anal cancer is very effective and cure rates are over 80 percent when diagnosed and treated early.

Cervical Dysplasias

Cervical dysplasia is the condition in which the squamous cells, or the glandular cells of the cervix, undergo abnormal transformation but have not become cancerous. Over 90 percent of cervical dysplasias occur in the squamous epithelium. The rest occur in the glandular epithelium. In this section, we will focus mainly on squamous epithelial cell abnormalities, which can be mild, moderate, or severe. Statistically, mild dysplasia is more likely to go away without any treatment than severe dysplasia, which has a higher probability of spreading to the adjacent tissues and becoming invasive cancer. As a general rule, it is *extremely uncommon* for cervical dysplasias to progress to cancer if they are properly treated and if women obtain their regular Pap test follow-up exams in a timely fashion.

Even to professionals, the term "cervical dysplasias" is confusing, as it is not always crystal clear which dysplasias will progress to cancer and which will not. The most important feature about dysplasia is that it is *limited* to the lining of the cervix (above a thin layer of tissue called the basement membrane) and has not invaded any of the underlying tissue. Once the basement membrane is broken and the underlying tissue is invaded, it ceases to be just dysplasia and has progressed to become invasive cancer.

Approximately 1 to 1.7 million American women are diagnosed with various stages of cervical dysplasias annually in the United States. Between 300,000 and 500,000 of them are precancerous lesions (Clifford et al. 2003). Cervical dysplasias can develop at any age, with ages 25 to 35 being the most common group affected. Over $2 billion is spent on diagnosing and treating cervical dysplasias in the United States alone.

The next section is devoted to a brief explanation, interpretation, and treatment of abnormal Pap tests. (We have already discussed the importance of obtaining Pap tests in the previous chapter.) Though this section could be somewhat technical, it will give you an idea of the complex nature of cervical dysplasias and the role the HPV vaccines play in preventing the various stages of dysplasia.

Classification of Abnormal Pap Tests

Since the days of Dr. George N. Papanicolaou, professionals in the medical field have been trying to communicate about cervical abnormalities and their standards of treatment in universal terms. In an effort to better correlate terminology and communications between the laboratory and the clinician, two systems were created. Both systems were designed

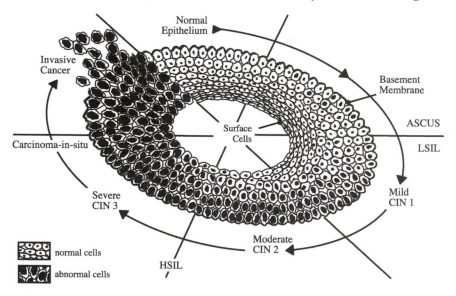

Figure 4.1 HPV Disease Progression: Normal Cells to Invasive Cancer
Illustrator: Zyamina Gorelik (c) 2008.

to describe a progression of cells from normal to low risk, low to high risk, and finally, high risk to malignant. These classification systems are the CIN system and the Bethesda classification for abnormal Pap smears.

The CIN System

The term "cervical intraepithelial neoplasia" (CIN) was introduced to present the concept of cervical neoplasia as a disease continuum. In the CIN system, the term "neoplasia" means "new growth," and the term "epithelium" means the surface layer of cells. Putting the terms together, "cervical intraepithelial neoplasia" means a new growth within the surface or the lining of the cervix. The different levels of CIN indicate the depth of the lining of the cervix that is invaded by abnormal cells. In other words, CIN is a histological classification that indicates the amount of tissue (a tissue is an organized collection of cells) that has been invaded by the abnormal cells.

- **CIN I:** Most of the cells show mild dysplasia; abnormal cells can be found in one-third of the lining of the cervix.
- **CIN II:** Most of the cells show moderate dysplasia; abnormal cells can be found in one-half to two-thirds of the lining of the cervix.
- **CIN III:** Most of the cells show severe dysplasia; abnormal cells can be found in more than two-thirds of the lining of the cervix and up to the full thickness of the lining.

When the cancer cells extend up to the full thickness of the basement membrane, the term "carcinoma *in situ*" is used. The word "carcinoma" means cancer, and "*in situ*" means "contained within." Therefore, "carcinoma *in situ*" means that the precancerous cells are still contained within the cervical lining and have not spread beyond the basement membrane. Carcinoma *in situ* is not invasive cancer, but it is the next-to-last step before invasive cancer. In the past, there was a tendency to treat carcinoma *in situ* like cancer, when in fact, it is still a dysplasia.

Persistent high-risk HPV infection is necessary for the development of all CIN II, CIN III, and invasive cancers. Statistically, only one in 10 to one in 30 HPV infections are associated with an abnormal Pap smear, and an even smaller proportion is associated with CIN II or CIN III. From a clinical standpoint, it is important to determine which intraepithelial neoplasias are less likely to progress to cancer, and which ones are more likely to progress to cancer *if not treated*. To emphasize this point, an even newer classification system, called the Bethesda System, was developed by the National Cancer Institute in 1989. This system classifies the cells as low grade (less likely to progress to cancer) or high grade (more likely to progress to cancer) *if not treated*. Therefore, the Bethesda system is a cytological (cytology is the study of cells) classification of abnormal cervical cells, whereas the CIN system is a histological (tissue) classification indicating the depth of tissue involvement.

Bethesda Classification for Abnormal Pap Smears

As noted earlier, the following terminologies can be confusing, but, as you will see later, it provides an important tool in understanding the HPV-related pathology:

- **ASCUS (atypical cells of undetermined significance):** This is the most common type of abnormal Pap smear—the category that, honestly, drives both clinicians and patients crazy. This means that some cells in the squamous epithelium of the cervix have undergone very mild changes either due to infection or irritation, but they are not abnormal enough to be called dysplasia. Of women who have ASCUS, 20–30 percent may have underlying severe or high grade lesions of the squamous epithelium (HSIL). Therefore, in order to further clarify which women in this category are at risk, ASCUS is further classified into ASC-US (unsatisfactory significance with lower or no risk) and ASC-H (cannot exclude a high-grade lesion). All cases of ASC-H require confirmation with further testing to evaluate the cervical abnormality.
- **AGC (atypical glandular cells):** AGC refers to abnormal cells that originate higher up in the cervical canal or uterus. AGC can indicate serious conditions such as cancer of the uterus. AGC results are considered rare, resulting in less than 1 percent of Pap smear results. Diagnosis of AGC warrants further testing to rule out a cancerous condition.
- **LSIL (low-grade squamous intraepithelial lesion):** An LSIL result means that there is mild dysplasia. HPV is considered to be the main cause of LSIL. Most cases of LSIL resolve spontaneously within two years. Depending on your age, your physician will direct you to further testing.
- **HSIL (high-grade squamous intraepithelial lesion):** HSIL is a more serious classification of cervical dysplasia. If left untreated, HSIL could lead to cervical cancer. HSIL comprises both CIN II and CIN III groups including carcinoma *in situ.* Beyond HSIL, the lesion is classified as an invasive squamous cell carcinoma. Seventy percent of women who have a HSIL lesion fall in the CIN II or CIN III category. Another 1 to 2 percent have invasive cancer. Therefore, a Pap smear result that has a report of HSIL will require further follow-up depending upon the severity of the lesion.
- **Invasive cancer:** Here the cancer has spread beyond the confines of the lining of the cervix and has invaded the tissue underlying the surface. Treatment for invasive cervical cancer is very different from treatment for cervical dysplasias. Cervical cancer will be discussed in detail later in this chapter.

> ☞ **In dysplasia, all of the abnormalities are confined to the cell lining of the cervix. They have not yet invaded the underlying tissue.**

Testing and Treatment Guidelines for Cervical Dysplasia

Once cervical dysplasia is confirmed, the treatment for it depends on the age of the patient and severity of the abnormality. As over 90 percent of HPV infections resolve spontaneously and rarely lead to cervical cancer in the younger age group, the American Association of Obstetricians and Gynecologists published in 2006 a new set of guidelines, which encourages a more "watch and wait" approach in treating cervical dysplasias among those women who are 20 and younger as compared to adults. However, depending on the severity of the dysplasia, one or more procedures may be employed. The following is a glossary of terms that are used when managing cervical dysplasias:

- **Colposcopy:** A device called the colposcope (a lighted, magnifying instrument) is used to directly examine the cervix and vagina under magnification.
- **Cervical biopsy:** A sample of tissue is taken from the abnormal lesion in the cervix.
- **Endocervical sampling or curettage:** This is a procedure where scrapings from the endocervical canal are obtained with the help of a curette (spoon-shaped instrument) and then tested for the presence of abnormal cells.
- **Endocervical assessment:** The endocervical canal is evaluated using a colposcope or endocervical sampling.
- **Loop Electrosurgical Excision Procedure (LEEP):** Electrical current is passed through a wire loop that is used to remove a very precise amount of abnormal tissue from the cervix.
- **Cryosurgery:** This method super-freezes and kills cancerous and precancerous cells.
- **Laser surgery:** A narrow beam of high-energy light is used to destroy precancerous and cancerous cells.
- **Conization:** A scalpel or a laser is used to remove a cone-shaped piece of the cervix containing the area with abnormal cells.
- **Excisional procedure:** A sample is obtained from the transformation zone and endocervical canal using LEEP or Conization.
- **Endometrial evaluation:** The lining of the uterus is evaluated, often with ultrasonography.
- **Ablative procedure:** Tissue is removed through radio wave frequency. Ablation therapy is frequently performed using a cryoprobe in which cold liquid nitrogen is passed through a hollow metal probe that is applied to the superficial tissue of the cervix. This freezes and destroys the dysplastic cells contained within the tissue.
- **Hysterectomy:** This is a major surgery that involves removal of the cervix and the uterus. A hysterectomy is sometimes done in selected cases of pre-invasive cancer.

Cervical Dysplasia and Pregnancy

In some women, the hormonal influences of pregnancy can trigger the progress of cervical dysplasias. As a general rule, cervical dysplasias are not treated during pregnancy due to the fear of accidentally starting early labor. Most cervical dysplasias, however, regress spontaneously after the

Table 4.2 Guidelines for the Management of Abnormal Pap Test Results

Pap test results	What the report means	Recommended follow-up for adults	Recommended follow-up for adolescents (20 and below)
ASCUS (atypical squamous cells of undetermined significance)	Unclear—some cells (squamous type) from outer layer of the cervix look abnormal; cause could be irritation, infection or HPV.	Several options available. If over the age of 30, HPV DNA testing. Between the ages of 21-30, repeat Pap in 6 months or proceed with HPV DNA testing.	No HPV DNA testing. Repeat Pap test in 12 months.
ASCUS (HPV negative)	Unclear abnormalities, but HPV negative.	Repeat Pap test in 12 months.	No HPV DNA testing. Follow ASCUS protocol.
ASCUS (HPV positive)	Unclear abnormalities, but HPV high-risk positive.	Colposcopy	No HPV DNA testing. Follow ASCUS protocol.
ASC-H (atypical squamous cells— high-grade lesion might be present)	Unclear significance—a high-grade lesion may be present, but the cell changes are too minor to be sure; this is equivalent to HSIL.	Refer for colposcopy and treat according to results.	Refer for colposcopy and treat according to results.
AGC (atypical glandular cells)	Some glandular cells from higher up in the lining of the cervical canal look abnormal; may indicate a condition that is more serious.	Colposcopy and treatment as recommended by your health-care provider.	Colposcopy and treatment as recommended by your health-care provider.

Term	Description		
LSIL (low-grade squamous intraepithelial lesion)	Squamous cells are minimally abnormal but usually not precancerous.	Colposcopy and treatment as recommended by your health-care provider.	Repeat Pap in 12 months and follow up as indicated.
HSIL (high-grade squamous intraepithelial lesion)—Precancer	Squamous cells are moderate to severely abnormal, and may turn into invasive cancer if not treated.	Colposcopy and endocervical biopsy. Treatment as indicated by biopsy results.	Colposcopy and endocervical biopsy. Treatment as indicated by biopsy results.
AIS (adenocarcinoma *in situ*)—Precancer	A precancerous lesion is found in the glandular tissue of the cervix.	Colposcopy and biopsy. Further treatment might include endocervical curettage and endometrial evaluation.	Colposcopy and biopsy. Further treatment might include endocervical curettage and endometrial evaluation.
Cancer	Cancer cells are present in the cervix.	Treatment options include surgery, radiation, and chemotherapy.	Treatment options include surgery, radiation, and chemotherapy.
CIN I	Abnormal cells are found up to one-third the depth of cervical lining.	Follow up with Pap/DNA testing as indicated by your health-care provider. Colposcopy for any abnormality.	Follow up with Pap as indicated by your health-care provider. Colposcopy for any abnormality.
CIN II	Abnormal cells are found up to two-thirds the depth of cervical lining.	Treatment as indicated by your health-care provider.	Follow up testing as indicated by your health-care provider.

| CIN III | Abnormal cells are found in the full thickness of the cervical lining. Carcinoma *in situ* is included in this category. | Will require testing and further treatment. | Will require testing and further treatment. |

Notes:

- Women 20 and younger do not require HPV DNA testing even for ASCUS, as most lesions will resolve spontaneously.
- Women of all ages with diagnosis of AGC (atypical glandular cells) require further testing with colposcopy, endocervical assessment, and possibly endometrial evaluation in order to rule out a cancerous condition.
- Women who have an LSIL lesion and are over the age of 20 require colposcopy. Women younger than 20 are followed up closely with annual Pap tests.
- CIN II and CIN III require close follow-up and treatment with ablative or excisional therapy in most cases.

Source: Based on the information provided by the American Society for Colposcopy and Cervical Pathology (ASCCP) and the American College of Obstetricians and Gynecologists (ACOG) consensus guidelines for the management of abnormal cervical cytological results (2006).

pregnancy has passed. If not, they have to be treated according to the guidelines set forth by the American Association of Obstetrics and Gynecologists after the delivery of the baby.

In the following section, we will discuss the disease of cervical cancer at length as it pertains to the HPV vaccines: who gets it, why, and whether the vaccines would reduce the incidence and death rates of cervical cancer in the United States and the world around.

Cervical Cancer

Cervical cancer is one of the most preventable types of cancer. At one time, cervical cancer was the leading cause of death among women in the United States. Today, according to the American Cancer Society, cervical cancer ranks as the 12th most common cancer among women in the United States. It comprises 1.6 percent of all cancers that develop in one year and 1.3 percent of all cancer deaths among females. Ninety-nine percent of cervical cancer infections are caused by HPV. Fortunately, the long interval between the acquisition of HPV infections and the development of invasive cervical cancer has allowed for the implementation of screening programs such as the Pap test to be largely responsible for the decline in cervical cancer death rates by 75 percent in the last 50 years. The death rate from cervical cancer continues to decline by nearly 4 percent every year.

Cervical cancer occurs when the abnormal cells break through the basement membrane of the cervical lining and invade the underlying tissue. Ninety percent of cervical cancers are squamous cell carcinomas that arise from the squamous cells on the ectocervix, and the remaining 10 percent are adenocarcinomas that arise from the glandular cells on the endocervix. More than half of the squamous cell carcinomas of the cervix are caused by HPV 16, followed by another 15–20 percent caused by HPV 18. Most adenocarcinomas are caused by HPV 18.

> ☞ Cervical cancer is very slow growing and one of the most preventable types of cancer. With regular Pap tests, cervical cancer can be prevented in almost all cases.

Cervical cancer is a very slow-growing cancer. It can take decades for an abnormal Pap smear to progress to invasive cancer. According to the National Cancer Institute, it is estimated that among women who develop cervical cancer, about 50 percent have never had a Pap test, and another 10 percent have not had a Pap test in the past five years. This glaring fact alone should be enough to motivate all women to get regular Pap smears as part of their medical routine.

Incidence and Prevalence

Statistics show that there are nearly 500,000 cases of cervical cancer annually around the world, with around 250,000 deaths resulting from it.

According to the United States Cancer Statistics 2004 Incidence and Mortality report, 11,892 women were diagnosed with cervical cancer in 2004, and 3,850 women died from the disease that same year in the United States. In addition, there were 250,726 women alive with a history of cancer of the cervix in the United States as of January 1, 2004. These numbers included women who were diagnosed with active disease and those who were cured of their disease.

The median age of diagnosis of cervical cancer is 47 years, and the median age at death is 57 years. Does cervical cancer discriminate among age, race, ethnicity, and region? The answer to all of these questions is a resounding YES.

Incidence Rate Based on Race and Ethnicity
Despite the consistent decline in cervical cancer deaths in the United States overall, high cervical cancer incidence rates and death rates have existed for decades in some ethnic populations. According to the National Cancer Institute, these groups include black women, Hispanic women, Native American women, Alaskan native women, and immigrant women from Asia. Among these high-risk groups, Hispanic women have the highest incidence rate for cervical cancer. The rate is over twice that of non-Hispanic Caucasian women. This is followed by black women, who develop this cancer about 50 percent more often than their non-Hispanic Caucasian counterparts. Table 4.3 gives information on cervical cancer incidence and cervical cancer deaths based on race and ethnicity.

From Table 4.3 one can see that Hispanic women had the highest incidence rate for cervical cancer (13.8/100,000). Black women had the second-highest incidence of getting cervical cancer (11.4/100,000). When it came to death rates from cervical cancer, black women (4.9/100,000) were more likely to die of cervical cancer than any other group. Hispanic women had the second-highest rate of deaths from cervical cancer (3.3/100.000), followed by women who are Native American/Native Alaskan (2.9/100,000), Asian/Pacific Islander (2.4/100,000), and white (2.3/100,000). Black women were found to have higher Pap test usage, but were less likely to come back for follow-up procedure after an abnormal Pap test result, either due to economic difficulties or poor knowledge of the disease consequences.

Geographical Differences in Cervical Cancer
Geographical variations also occur. Black women from the rural South (Hall et al. 2004), Hispanic women from near the Texas-Mexico border (Coronado et al. 2004), and white women from Appalachia (410 mostly rural counties in 13 states extending from New York to Mississippi) are the most affected within their subgroups (Yabroff et al. 2005). Even though the overall incidence of cervical cancer among white women is the lowest, those native to the Appalachian region have among the

Table 4.3 Incidence Rates, Trends, and Death Rates from Cervical Cancer (approximate) in the United States

Race or ethnicity	Number of cases/year 2000–2004	Incidence rates/ 100,000 women 2000–2004	*Decline* in inci- dence trends from mid-1990s–2004	Deaths/year 2000–2004	Death rates/ 100,000 women 2000–2004	*Decline* in death trends from mid-1990s–2004
All	11,892	8.7	3.7%	3850	2.6%	3.7%
African American	1866	11.4	3.7%	789	4.9%	4.7%
Asian/Pacific Islander	479	8.0	5.9%	131	2.4%	4.5%
Hispanic/Latino	1839	13.8	3.6%	430	3.3%	3.3%
American Indian/ Alaskan	88	6.6	Remained level	31	4.0%	Remained level
White	7620	8.5	Very small decline	2469	2.3%	Remained level

Source: Based on information from United States Cancer Statistics Working Group. *United States Cancer Statistics: 2004 Incidence and Mortality,* Atlanta (GA): Department of Health and Human Services, Centers for Disease Control and Prevention, and Surveillance, Epidemiology, and End Results (SEER)—Program National Cancer Institute.

highest cervical cancer incidence rates (around 10.7/100,000). About
65 percent of Appalachia is rural, and its population is generally
white and poor with low educational levels. It was found that those
who were living below the poverty line and had very low rates of higher
education had very high rates of cancer. These regions include the eastern
parts of Kentucky and northern parts of Tennessee and West Virginia.
This region as a whole also has a high prevalence of other cancer risk
factors, such as tobacco use, physical inactivity, and inadequate access to
medical care.

The geographical distribution of cervical cancer around the world also
varies. It is lowest in countries where there are well-established and
successfully run Pap test screening programs. For example, the incidence
rate of cervical cancer in women in the United Kingdom is around
8/100,000 and in Canada is 8.4/100,000. Approximately 70 to 80 percent of
women in the United Kingdom and 65–91 percent in Canada (a figure that
varies according to age) are regularly screened with Pap smears, according
to their respective National Census Bureaus. Recent surveys in the United
States between 1998 and 2000 show that approximately two-thirds of
women born after 1930 report having been screened in the previous year,
and approximately 85 percent within the previous three years.

In contrast, cervical cancer is much more prevalent in countries where
there are no well-established cervical screening programs. For example,
the prevalence of cervical cancer for women in Brazil is 18.6/100,000
and in Thailand is 15.6 /100,000.

Cervical Cancer Trends in Foreign-born Women in the United States
Cervical cancer mortality is dependent on a complex network of factors, and the continued influx of immigrants to the United States is one
of them. According to the mortality data derived from the National
Center for Health Statistics, between 1985 and 1996, incidence and death
rates from cervical cancer in foreign-born women increased, whereas they
decreased for U.S.-born women. Socioeconomic and cultural barriers
were cited as some of the causative factors. Experts have also observed
that the sexual behavior of the male partner in certain cultures plays an
important role in predicting a minority woman's risk for contracting
cervical cancer—more so, even, than her own sexual history.

To give an example, cervical cancer rates among women in Latin
America are three to four times higher than the rates found among
all women in the United States. In order to understand the underlying cause of these high rates, a study was done among 971 Hispanic
women between the ages of 18 and 47 in the United States from 1992 to
1995. It compared women who were born in Mexico and immi-
grated to the United States to Mexican American women born in the
United States. The study showed that even though the women born in
Mexico had a low sexual behavior risk profile, meaning they had fewer

sexual partners and were older at the age of their first intercourse when compared to Mexican American women born in the United States, women born in Mexico had a significantly higher rate of HPV infections when compared to their United States–born counterparts. This increased risk for HPV infections and, hence, cervical cancer among Hispanic women (even though this study was biased toward women of Mexican origin from the lower socioeconomic class) was attributed to the sexual history of their male partners. It was found that even though Mexican American women born in the United States had more sexual partners, their partners used barrier methods such as condoms at a much higher rate when compared to the partners of women who were born in Mexico. In Mexico, male "maschismo" is expressed sexually through having multiple partners, casual sexual contacts, and unprotected sex, all of which start at an early age and may continue after marriage. In addition, frequenting female prostitutes is an accepted way of life among many Mexican men, regardless of their socioeconomic status. All of these factors can increase the risk of HPV infections among their female sexual partners. Further research, however, is needed to corroborate these findings (Giuliano et al. 1999).

Healthy People, a national initiative established to improve the health of Americans, has set goals to have no more than two deaths per 100,000 from cervical cancer by 2010. In order to accomplish these goals, public officials will have to include

> ☞ Poverty, poor access to health care, poor levels of education, and being foreign born are factors that play a bigger role than geography in the incidence and death rates from cervical cancer in the United States.

more effective strategies in reducing the racial, ethnic, and regional disparities. They should also take into consideration the increased statistics for cervical cancer incidence in the foreign-born community. Awareness programs such as culturally sensitive cancer education, prevention, and screening measures should also be instituted in addition to addressing the global burden of the disease.

Symptoms of Cervical Cancer

Early stages of cervical cancer usually do not exhibit any outward symptoms. Sometimes, an unusual vaginal discharge can be a sign of cervical cancer. Such a discharge may include bloody spotting or light bleeding and may occur between menstrual cycles. Once the cancer becomes invasive, the most common symptom is abnormal bleeding, which may occur between menstrual periods or after sexual intercourse. Periods may be heavier and last longer than usual. Postmenopausal bleeding can also be an indication of cervical cancer.

Staging

Staging is the process that defines how far a cancer has spread. Staging is an important measure because it helps tailor the right treatment plan (see Table 4.4). On average, 51 percent of cervical cancer cases are diagnosed while the cancer is still confined to the primary site (localized stage); 34 percent are diagnosed after the cancer has spread beyond the confines of the cervix but is still confined within the pelvis (the space that contains the urogenital organs); 9 percent are diagnosed after the cancer has already metastasized (to a distant site such as the lung or breast).

Five-Year Survival Rate

The five-year survival rate refers to the proportion of people who are still alive five years after positive diagnosis. Doctors often use this term when discussing the prognosis of a particular stage of cancer. The reason to choose five years as a significant milestone comes from the empirical data that shows the chances for cervical cancer to recur after five years of treatment is very small. The overall five-year relative survival rate for cervical cancer in the years 1996–2003, in the areas surveyed by the National Cancer Institute in the United States, was 71.6 percent. Five-year relative survival rates by race were: 72.9 percent for white women and 62.2 percent for black women.

Treatment

Table 4.4 gives an overview of the various stages, survival rates, and treatment modalities used in the different stages of cervical cancer.

Pregnancy and Cervical Cancer

When cervical cancer is diagnosed during pregnancy, treatment decisions will depend upon the stage of the cancer and the stage of the pregnancy. If the cancer is diagnosed during the first trimester, painful decisions such as terminating the pregnancy may have to be considered, as cancer treatment can harm the unborn baby significantly, and if treatment is not carried out, the mother's life may be in jeopardy. On the other hand, for cancer found during the third trimester, treatment can sometimes be delayed until after the baby is born.

HPV VACCINES

Two new vaccines against the human papillomavirus are now available. Both have shown to be highly effective against certain strains of HPV in clinical trials. One (*Gardsil*, by Merck) has already been approved by the Food and Drug Administration, and the other (*Cervarix*, by Glaxo-SmithKline) is scheduled to be licensed soon in the United States.

Table 4.4 Cervical Cancer: Staging, Survival Rate, and Treatment

Stage	What it means	Available treatment options	Five-year survival rates after treatment
0	Carcinoma *in situ*	LEEP, conization	**Nearly 100%**
I	The cancer has broken through the basement membrane but has not spread anywhere else.		80%–>95%
IA	The area of invasion is less than 5 mm deep and less than 7 mm wide.	Hysterectomy, internal radiation therapy, conization, trachelectomy	96%–99%
IB	The area of invasion is greater than 5 mm deep and 7 mm wide. The lesion is still confined to the cervix, but can be seen without a microscope.	Internal and external radiation therapy, radical hysterectomy with lymph node dissection, followed by radiation and chemotherapy, radiation and chemotherapy alone.	80%–90%
II	Here the cancer has spread beyond the confines of the cervix but has not spread up to the pelvic wall.		75%–78%
IIA	Here the cancer has invaded the upper part of the vagina.	Usually treated the same way as Stage IB.	Same
IIB	Here the cancer has spread to the tissues adjacent to the cervix but has not invaded the side walls of the pelvis.	Internal and external radiation therapy combined with chemotherapy.	Same
III	The cancer has spread to the lower one-third of the vagina and may include spread to the pelvic wall.	Same as stage IIB. Treatment is usually more intensive and takes much longer. Also survival rates are poorer.	47%–50%

IIIA	The cancer has spread to the lower third of the vagina but not to the pelvic wall.		Same
IIIB	The cancer extends to the pelvic walls and or blocks one or both the ureters (the tubes that carry urine from the kidneys to the bladder.		Same
IV	This is the most advanced stage of the cancer.	Same as stage III, but with even longer and more intensive treatment with worse five-year survival rates.	**15%–30%**
IVA	The cancer has spread to the adjacent organs such as the bladder and the rectum.		20%–30%
IVB	The cancer has spread to distant organs beyond the pelvic area such as the lungs or the liver.	Cancer is usually not considered curable. Keeping the patient comfortable is the priority at this stage of the disease.	15%–20%

Source: Based on information from the American Cancer Society.

The advent of these two vaccines is considered by many experts as one of the greatest advances in women's medical history in recent times. They believe that the vaccines could have a dramatic effect in changing the statistics of cervical cancer. This, perhaps, could be very true in developing countries where cancer rates are high. But, how about in a country like the United States where cervical cancer rates are already low and where the population at greatest risk is the women with low cervical cancer screening rates? Will the vaccine be able to circumvent the challenges presented by these populations such as those residing in rural areas and inner cities, ethnic minority women, immigrant women, older women, and the uninsured?

Federally sponsored programs, such as the National Breast and Cervical Cancer Early Detection Program (NBCCEDP), that provide screening services for underserved women in the United States have met with challenges to bring the success of screening programs to these populations equally. Unfortunately, it is highly likely that this same group may also be left behind as the HPV vaccine is administered.

In my opinion, the vaccines can help reduce the cervical cancer rates *only* if they can target this same group of women who do not obtain or cannot be accessed for regular Pap smears today. Unless this demographic, which is experiencing a disproportionate burden of the disease, is effectively reached with the vaccination and screening programs, the introduction of the vaccines will only have a minimal effect on changing the cervical cancer rates in this country. The American Cancer Society is also in agreement with this perspective.

> The vaccine holds a remarkable potential to change cervical mortality rates, but, unless it targets the same group of women who are not receiving their Pap tests today, the impact of the vaccine will be curtailed.

Strong public will and political support, coupled with women taking responsibility for themselves, can, we hope, bring this ugly chapter of cervical cancer to a satisfactory close. Cervical cancer is a unique public health challenge and is an indicator of a larger health-care disparity that includes health-care access, cultural and ethical issues, and the delivery of public health education. Effectively addressing the issue of cervical cancer can also provide a model for a host of other diseases that stem from sheer health-care disparities such as heart disease and HIV.

As we draw this chapter to a close, let me leave you with some food for thought:

1. If cervical cancer rates are so low in the United States and other developed countries, should women who are educated, health conscious, and able to access regular cervical screening require the vaccine at all?
2. Does the vaccine have any benefits other than preventing cervical cancer? If so, what are they?
3. Why should only females and not males be vaccinated; especially when HPV is a sexually transmitted disease?

These are some of the compelling questions that will be discussed in the ensuing chapters. But, before that, let us turn our attention to the next chapter, which covers a very important but often neglected aspect of HPV infections: the emotional impact of HPV.

Key Facts

- Warts are the most common and benign manifestations of genital HPV infections.
- Most cervical dysplasias resolve spontaneously. Very few progress to invasive cancer.
- Cervical cancer is the most serious manifestation of HPV infections.
- Cervical cancer is more common among women who are from low socioeconomic backgrounds and those who do not seek or have access to regular Pap smears.
- More than half the women who had cervical cancer did not get a Pap smear in the previous five years.

5

EMOTIONAL ASPECTS AND PREVENTION OF HPV: SHAME, BLAME, AND ABSENCE OF CURE

Myth: Raising public awareness that HPV is a sexually transmitted disease will increase scrutiny of women's morality and heighten their levels of anxiety about the disease.

Fact: Raising public awareness about the nature of HPV infections and their prevalence will actually *decrease* the level of anxiety associated with the disease.

The human papillomavirus has outsmarted humans and the field of medicine for many, many generations. The virus invades the human body with great ease and then exerts a strong and permanent hold, bringing with it varying degrees of medical, emotional, and sexual upheaval. Its three-way threat—a silent infection, an incurable infection, and an infection that can cause cancer—can lead to tremendous emotional turmoil in many men and women. One would think that, in the age of modern medicine and with the advent of antiviral drugs, HPV would be a thing of the past. Not so. One would also think that, because the virus is so common and can cause a potentially serious infection, people would be extremely knowledgeable about the do's and don'ts to minimize exposure. Also not so. Unfortunately, the disconnect between the common prevalence of HPV and the lack of awareness among the public is overwhelming. This is not unusual when one considers the general tendency in our society to avoid public discourse and education on any topic that can be considered taboo by the political and religious establishments. The hope is that it will somehow go away so that we do not have to deal with it. For example, early in the AIDS epidemic, the prevalent theory was that only gay men got AIDS.

Some prominent leaders even came out and said that AIDS was God's revenge against an abhorrent lifestyle and the gay community's sins. It was only natural, then, that governmental support for AIDS research was less than enthusiastic. Only when AIDS began to spread to the larger heterosexual population did the country begin to pay more attention. Ryan White, a young white heterosexual teenager from Middle America, contracted AIDS in the mid-1980s, and he became an incredibly dignified poster child for the AIDS virus. Ryan suffered from a blood disorder called hemophilia since birth, and he required frequent blood transfusions. He contracted AIDS from one of these transfusions. His public school in Kokomo, Indiana, expelled him because they felt that he would be a health risk to the other students. His family fought with the school board to keep him in school. Unfortunately, Ryan died of AIDS shortly afterward. Suddenly, there was a national outcry and a call for "all hands on deck" to stop the ravages of the disease before it was too late.

Most HPV infections cause no symptoms and clear up on their own. However, being diagnosed with the disease can take a tremendous emotional toll on a patient and his or her partner. In addition, health-care providers' failure to provide adequate emotional support and clear information on the psychological aspects of the disease have left a significant proportion of women and some men worrying needlessly about having the virus.

Psychologically, an HPV diagnosis for a woman can bring a sense of vulnerability, loneliness, and anger at herself and her partner (Clarke et al. 1996). Externally disfiguring symptoms such as warts evoke an overbearing sense of disgust and anxiety in men and women of all ages. The infected individual may feel guilty, have a sense of diminished social worth as a future partner, and think that his or her sexual life has come to a grinding halt (Campion et al. 1988). This, in turn, could lead to self-inflicted blame and problems with sexuality. Those in monogamous relationships fear their partner's reaction and potential questions surrounding their fidelity. This could all eventually lead to a "free for all" blame game that is pernicious in what once was a beautiful relationship. Patients also have to deal with emotions of shame and guilt and associated problems with their own sexuality.

While blame and possibilities of rejection loom in the minds of younger women with genital warts, the diagnosis of abnormal Pap smears brings on a completely new set of emotions. In addition to shame, guilt, and stigma it also raises the fear of cancer (Mast et al. 2001). Lack of knowledge about low-risk versus high-risk HPV types also brings about unnecessary worries. In older women, the probability of developing cervical cancer and the disruption of the family routine seem to be the foremost concerns.

It is now clear that the diagnosis of HPV can bring with it emotions of shame, stigmatization, alienation, and fear. However, women with more knowledge about the disease process can lower their anxiety levels. While no amount of knowledge can prevent the overwhelming surge of fear and emotion that many women feel when they are initially diagnosed and informed about a sexually transmitted disease that has the potential to cause cancer, presenting them with important information about the disease can help ease their worries. From my personal experience of having to convey difficult and unfortunate news to patients on numerous occasions, I have found that sound medical advice, when given without addressing the patient's emotional status first, falls on deaf ears. The patient's anxiety level is so high that the very information that can actually be helpful in reducing their negative emotions associated with the diagnosis is often misinterpreted, leaving no chance that it will lower the psychological impact. Another unfortunate fact that works against patients is that health-care providers are often hard-pressed for time, and they are unable to provide the emotional support that is needed on a long-term basis after the diagnosis of HPV (Guy 1993). One of my own patients who was diagnosed with an abnormal Pap smear over the summer by her doctor returned to school in the fall and said, "When I was diagnosed with HPV, my doctor came in and told me that I had HPV and went on about what procedure I was going to undergo and how I should be followed up. But she never stopped to find out how I *felt* about the diagnosis. I freaked out and was completely oblivious to most of her recommendations. My mother later told me that the doctor had been very thorough in explaining the disease process, the medical treatment, and follow-up schedules."

The psychological impact of an HPV diagnosis can vary from person to person. Personally, I find it best to address the questions and concerns of emotionally traumatized patients over a series of visits, depending on the mental state and needs of the patient. This not only allows time for the patients to acknowledge their diagnosis, but it also helps them process the information more clearly with a calmer state of mind. Follow-up visits also help in addressing any questions that may have arisen in the interim and give the clinician the opportunity to educate the patient in self-care and prevention.

Since addressing the emotional aspects of HPV is of prime importance, the following section deals with those issues in more detail. Even though they are primarily targeted toward women, men who have HPV or have partners with HPV can also benefit from the ensuing discussion.

The emotional, sexual, and preventive issues of HPV can be addressed in the following three phases:

Phase I: Crisis intervention—focusing mainly on shame, blame, and partner issues.

Phase II: Continued support—in issues related to emotions, sex and sexuality.

Phase III: Self-care and prevention—divided into:
- Primary prevention
- Secondary prevention

- Tertiary prevention
- Boosting the immune system through holistic healing

PHASE I—CRISIS INTERVENTION

In the first phase, or crisis intervention, the patient is often in a state of mental shock and mild trauma. Her first thoughts regard issues surrounding her current partner's possible infidelity and a reflection on her own sexual practices. This stage requires a lot of hand-holding, anticipation, and sympathy toward the patient's feelings. The patient will have a multitude of questions that will typically include how and when she contracted the HPV, who gave it to her, how she should talk to her partner, and should her partner be checked. A typical sample of the questions that the patient will have is shown in the sidebar. The overriding principle to adopt here is to be truthful and firm, yet caring and diplomatic—understandably, this is easier said than done.

- Who gave it to me?
- When did I get HPV?
- Why me?
- Should I tell my partner?
- What should I tell my partner? And how should I do it?
- Will this ruin our relationship?
- Should my partner be checked?
- Should I tell my previous partners? If so, how far back?
- What should I tell my future partners?

Who Gave It to Me?

This is a difficult question to answer because the virus can remain dormant for several years. But, if you have been in a monogamous relationship and have *never* had sexual contact with anyone else before, then it is reasonable to say that your current partner has given it to you. However, your being diagnosed with HPV now is *not* a reflection on your current partner's fidelity to you at any time in your relationship. He or she could have contracted it from a previous partner and not have even known about it. Similarly, if you have had sexual contact prior to your current relationship, then you may have carried the virus for a long time without even knowing that you have it.

When Did I Get HPV?

You can sometimes trace the onset of infection based on the symptoms that you are manifesting. The incubation period for genital warts is usually three to four months. So, if you have had the same partner for the past 6 months, chances are that he or she gave it to you. On the other hand, if you have had sexual contact with your current partner for less than a month and were in a sexual relationship with someone else before that, then there is a greater chance that the previous partner transmitted the virus to you. However, none of this can be stated with any certainty, simply because of the natural history of the virus. For other clinical manifestations such as abnormal Pap smears, the incubation period is much longer (average of 24 months), but varies widely. Also, most of these lesions clear up on their own in about 18–24 months. As difficult as it may seem, the important thing here is not to play the blame game, but to get both you and your partner educated about HPV and checked by your respective health-care providers.

Why Me?

HPV is a very prevalent infection. Even having sexual contact just once (with or without sexual intercourse) or having only one partner can put you at risk. Obviously, your chances of harboring the infection increase if you engage in high-risk sexual behavior, such as having unprotected sex or sex with multiple partners. It is also possible to get HPV from sexual contact without intercourse such as foreplay and nonsexual contact such as autoinoculation (through fingernails), the chances of which are greatly enhanced if you have a weakened immune system.

Should I Tell My Partner?

This is always a tough question to answer. Even though some use secrecy as a tool and refuse to disclose the diagnosis because it makes them feel inferior or insecure, I believe honesty is the best policy. Most patients manage the information based upon how much risk is involved in their relationship. As one of my patients said, "If I were not physically intimate, I would not see the need to share the information. But if I were to get sexually involved, then I would let that person know beforehand."

My suggestion to my patients is that there is more than one reason it would be a good idea to talk to their partners about HPV infections. If you wait until you get to the point of initiating sexual activity, chances are you are both already emotionally involved with each other and it may seem like you "baited" or trapped your partner before informing him or her of the issue. If, at that time, both of you decide not to proceed with your relationship, the emotional toll will be more severe for both of you. However, if you inform your partner earlier, the toll is decidedly less, and both of you know exactly where you stand with each other. Immediate honesty is always the best policy in this case. If both of you decide to proceed after this, you can be assured that you will have an open relationship based on trust between the two of you—the very best kind of relationship you can hope for.

Another patient said, "Even though I am not sure if I really want to tell him, I cannot go to bed with him knowing that I am withholding something from him. This will ruin my intimacy with him."

My response to this concern is that if you are already sexually involved with your partner but choose to keep your diagnosis a secret, you will be ultimately sacrificing a significant source of support—someone who could eventually help you with your self-esteem and reassurance. By communicating your fears and concerns, you will actually be able to get closer to your partner.

What Should I Tell My Partner? And, How Should I Do It?

Disclosure can bring anxiety and fear-ridden moments. But by opening up to a partner and talking about the HPV diagnosis, you are showing that you respect and care about him or her. Ultimately, the outcome of disclosure will depend on the degree of trust and communication in your relationship. Having prior knowledge about HPV will also help both of you cope with the infection in a more objective manner. If you are unsure about how to approach this, it may be advisable to schedule an appointment for both of you with your health-care provider so that he or she can answer any questions you have and recommend a course of action to take. Your health-care provider may be able to blunt or even prevent any emotional finger pointing and help you both concentrate on moving forward.

Here is an example of how one of my patients brought up the subject with her partner: "I really want to have a very personal chat with you before we engage in any form of sexual activity. I feel I can trust you and I thought you should know something about me before we get any closer. Last year, I found out that I had genital HPV. I am being followed up by my doctor. HPV is very prevalent, but it is a silent infection. The majority of HPV infections clear without a person even realizing that she is infected. Anyway, I think it will be a good idea for you to hear this from your doctor and get checked out too."

On the other hand, if you are talking to a partner with whom you have already had an intimate sexual relationship then you could say something like: "I just wanted to let you know that my doctor has diagnosed me with HPV. Apparently, HPV infection is very common and it is possible that you may also have it. Either I got it from you or you got it from me, we'll never know. This really does not matter in our relationship because we must have passed it back and forth several times between the two of us. What would help at this point is for you to also talk to your doctor."

Will This Ruin Our Relationship?

Once you have tested the waters and approached the subject, one of several things can happen: Your partner can either acknowledge that he or she understands and reassures you that the relationship is too important for this to come between the two of you, or he or she may react with anger and show disdain. This will once again depend on prior knowledge about the disease, how long you both have known each other, and how much you are committed to one another. In any event, be prepared to have some information about the topic on hand. This can help alleviate some stress and tension that may arise from revealing the diagnosis. Be confident and encourage him or her to follow up with a trusted health-care professional.

One of my patients in her mid-thirties once said to me "I don't want to hide anything from him. I know he loves me enough that if I explained the nature of the HPV infections, he will accept the condition without judging me." In intimate and long-term relationships, the fear of jeopardizing your partner's health is of primary concern. Nonetheless, a diagnosis of HPV in a stable relationship can create some alterations in the future dynamics of the relationship. One always wishes for a positive outcome and the continuation of a good relationship. One of my male patients once told me, "I want to do the right thing. So far, our relationship has been based on honesty, and I surely don't want to hurt her health. If she has further questions, I will have her talk to you."

Should My Partner Be Checked?

In a long-term relationship, you and your partner have probably passed the virus back and forth several times (the so-called "ping-pong effect"). In such cases, testing is redundant because there is a very good chance that your partner also has the virus. It will be best for you to use condoms or other barrier methods until your active lesions clear. Your partner's health-care provider will examine and advise him or her further if necessary. If you are infected together, then you have to heal together. It is as simple as that.

Should I Tell My Previous Partners? If So, How Far Back?

HPV is a tricky virus. It is tough to decide how far back to go in informing previous sexual partners. As a general rule, going back about 24 months seems reasonable, as the average incubation period for HPV to cause abnormal Pap smears is about that long if the infection has not already cleared itself. The incubation period for genital warts is much shorter. Informing previous partners also helps them to take extra precautions, such as consistent use of condoms, in curtailing the spread of infection.

What Should I Tell My Future Partners?

As discussed earlier, if you are going to be talking to a new partner, it might be a good idea to get to know your partner first and find out about his or her personal values before the presence of an STI becomes a factor in the progression of your relationship. This also gives the partner the time to gauge whether he or she would like to persist with the relationship once you have disclosed your condition. But, at any cost, NEVER wait until after you have had sex. The issue of HPV may get entwined in feelings of anger and mistrust, and the relationship could end unpleasantly.

After addressing these questions, the initial doctor's visit can usually be concluded. I send my patient home with written information about HPV basics for her to share with her partner and some added information about the specific type of HPV infection that she has. I then recommend that I see her again in one week for follow-up.

PHASE II—CONTINUED SUPPORT

The second phase deals with providing the patient continued support and facilitating her coping with the disease in an objective and constructive manner. A patient who is severely traumatized by her new diagnosis may typically say, "I feel so ashamed because I have an STI (McCaffery et al. 2006). I cannot eat, sleep, or talk to my best friend about it. I am afraid she will think I am dirty. I feel I have to live with this secret for the rest of my life because I don't want to be rejected by the people who love me. I feel there is something wrong with me. I don't like this feeling."

Emotions resulting from the diagnosis vary anywhere from total acceptance to heightened anxiety to devastation, depending on the patient's attitude toward the diagnosis. A condition becomes stigmatizing only when another individual shuns, criticizes, or looks at the person with disdain as a result of their condition. Treating a patient in a way that causes her shame is akin to being highly insensitive and/or judgmental when the patient is most vulnerable.

During this phase, I ask my patients to fill out a questionnaire that I have designed to aid me in addressing their most pressing issues in a more systematic manner (see Table 5.1). This also helps me gauge the extent of their emotional turmoil: if it seems that their worries have gone beyond the "normal and expectable" realm of reaction, then it allows me to decide if they would benefit from referral to a counselor for continuing support. Most patients have several questions regarding sex and sexuality that they are willing to put down on paper rather than broach the subject directly with their health-care provider. The written survey attempts to extract the honest and forthright feelings of the patient, which then allows me to more accurately gauge the course of treatment to prescribe her.

The majority of HPV patients—two-thirds to three-fourths—experience to varying degrees the feelings and concerns listed in Table 5.1. A few are not concerned about the infection and are quite capable of moving on without too much trepidation. For all patients, these symptoms get better with time. The time frame in which they continue to have these feelings also varies with patients, but it is not unusual for some of them to feel this way for up to one year. During treatment, some of the more common

Table 5.1 Questionnaire to Gauge Emotional Impact of HPV Diagnosis

Statement	Strongly agree	Agree	Disagree	Strongly disagree
I feel more vulnerable.				
I am always preoccupied with my diagnosis.				
I have frequent mood problems (anger, depression, shame, guilt, blame, etc.).				
I am very afraid that I will develop cancer.				
My sexual drive has decreased.				
I fear rejection.				
I am apprehensive of future relationships.				
I fear that I will have trouble getting pregnant.				
I am not concerned with the diagnosis of HPV at all since it is so prevalent.				

questions that patients ask deal with middle- to long-term issues such as length of treatment, transmission to spouse or partner, and the ability to get pregnant and have children. A sample of questions pertaining to such issues is provided in the sidebar.

- Will my sex life change?
- Will I be able to transmit and reinfect my partner after treatment?
- Will my partner have to use condoms forever?
- Is there any risk to having oral sex?
- How about anal sex?
- Will I have any trouble getting pregnant?
- Can I transmit the virus to my child during pregnancy?

The patient has overcome the initial shock and is now looking for answers that will determine how she plans for the middle to long term. Some of the answers to these questions may affect the rest of her life and will determine the path she takes that best balances what she needs to do from a medical standpoint and how that complements her wishes to fulfill her own desires.

There is no doubt that the greatest impact of HPV falls on the sexual aspects of the disease (Clarke et al. 1996). Before the patient can educate or convince her partner, the all-important first step is to establish her own comfort level and give herself a good foundation of knowledge. The following are my answers to some of most frequently asked questions pertaining to sexual issues.

Will My Sex Life Change?

The presence of any kind of sexually transmitted infection including HPV generally necessitates a degree of adjustment and accommodation in the sexual relationship. For example, in a relationship where there were no barrier methods used in the past, the couple may now decide to use condoms until the active lesions have cleared. Some couples may decide to stop having intercourse altogether until the infection has cleared or until they both feel comfortable to resume sexual activity. The key thing is to pace yourselves and get comfortable with the new dynamics. You need to be fully ready both physically and mentally to resume sexual activity for it to be mutually fulfilling and satisfactory.

Will I Be Able to Transmit and Re-infect My Partner after Treatment?

HPV is a silent disease. Even after treatment, it can hide in your body for years and resurface itself anytime. Therefore it is not easy to provide a clear cut "yes" or "no" answer to the question.

Infections such as chlamydia, gonorrhea, and herpes cause inflammation of tissues, thereby facilitating the spread of HPV. Chemical irritations with douches and creams can also cause skin irritation. Mental stress can derail the immune system and lead to recurrences. If both you and your partner follow healthy lifestyles, recurrences are less apt to follow. One should be aware that active lesions carry the greatest risk of transmission.

Will My Partner Have to Use Condoms Forever?

Studies have now shown that condoms can reduce the transmission of HPV by 70 percent. Even though HPV can spread without sexual intercourse, condoms also prevent other STIs.

A trickier question is what you would do in a long-term relationship such as marriage in which you and your partner have not used condoms in years. In such a situation, using condoms would be redundant. You and your partner have both been infected by now by the same virus (due to the ping-pong effect), so condoms are not going to be very beneficial. I would, however, recommend using them when active lesions are being treated and until they have cleared clinically. When in doubt, always consult your health-care provider for advice.

Is There Any Risk to Having Oral Sex?

If you are having oral sex, here is what you should know:

- HPV can be transmitted to the mouth from someone who has genital HPV.
- Even though HPV can cause oral cancer, the association is not as strong as HPV to cervical and anal cancers.
- Types 6, 11, 16, and 18 can be transmitted to the mouth, but rarely cause oral warts and oral cancer.
- Condoms and dental dams can minimize transmission of HPV.

How About Anal Sex?

Anal sex carries a higher rate of transmission for STIs than vaginal sex. It is *always* a good idea to use condoms during anal sex regardless of whether one has HPV or not. It is best to talk to your health-care provider about anal sex so that he or she can assess your individual risks and advise you appropriately.

Will I Have Any Trouble Getting Pregnant?

HPV infections should not cause any problems with fertility or pregnancy. However, the more abnormal the Pap smear is, the more invasive the procedures for treatment are. Procedures such as a LEEP (electrosurgical excision procedure) may be required to cut away abnormal cervical tissue with a heated thin wire loop electrode. LEEP can sometimes weaken the cervix and cause miscarriages. Abnormal Pap smears detected during pregnancy are watched closely and preferably treated after delivery of the baby.

Can I Transmit the Virus to My Child during Pregnancy?

The answer is yes, but it is very rare. HPV lesions usually do not cause harm to the fetus. There is, however, a rare condition called "recurrent respiratory papillamatosis (RRP)," which is a benign condition, but it can cause symptoms of respiratory distress in children. Children can also get another rare disease called "conjunctival papillomas" in their eye. The papillomas have to be removed. RRP is discussed in greater detail in Chapter 7.

PHASE III—SELF-CARE AND PREVENTION

Being knowledgeable about the disease promotes optimal self-care and prevention. The only sure way to accomplish this is through EDUCATION.

At this point, I would like to share the results of a study that was conducted by Jo Waller and associates at the Cancer Research UK Health Behavior Unit, Department of Epidemiology and Public Health University College, London. They conducted a Web-based study among 811 female students to whom information about HPV was provided. Even though this was a small study, it was one of very few that have been conducted to show that raising awareness about HPV was important. In this study, the students were asked to imagine that they had tested positive for HPV and the relationship between their degree of knowledge about HPV and their associated feelings of shame, stigma, and anxiety was measured. Results showed that there were great differences observed among students in their emotional reactions to imagining testing positive to HPV. The overall conclusions of the study were:

- Knowledge that infection had a high rate of prevalence was associated with lower levels of stigma, shame, and anxiety.
- Knowledge that HPV is sexually transmitted was associated with highest levels of stigma and shame, but not anxiety.
- Women who knew that HPV is sexually transmitted but not aware of the high prevalence rate displayed the highest levels of stigma and shame.
- Receiving a positive HPV result is associated with higher anxiety than simply having an abnormal smear result.
- Knowing that HPV is highly prevalent reduces the level of shame and thereby somehow normalizes the infection. Research shows that an infection perceived to be common is judged to be less serious than those perceived to be rare.

The following set of questions are usually posed by my patients regarding self-care and prevention. Many are interested in knowing if there are "natural ways" to prevent and treat HPV infections.

- How long will I have this infection?
- Is there a cure for HPV infections?
- How can I prevent HPV infections?
- What is the role of vaccinations in preventing and treating HPV infections?
- Are there any natural ways to fight HPV infections?

How Long Will I Have This Infection?

Due to the natural history of the virus, it is hard to tell how long infections last. The clinical manifestation of HPV such as warts and abnormal Pap smears can be treated, but there is no guarantee that the treatment equals a complete cure. As the virus can lay dormant for years, the test of cure is difficult to assess. As a general rule of thumb, however, the incubation period for external genital warts is around three months (from a minimum of six weeks to possibly around eight months). In the case of abnormal Pap smears, the time frame is 12–24 months. With a healthy immune system, most infections clear up within one to two years.

In a minority of the cases where women continue to have persistent infections, more serious consequences such as precancerous and cancerous lesions can occur if not screened and treated regularly.

Is There a Cure for HPV Infections?

Unfortunately, because HPV is a viral infection like the common cold, there is no known method to cure HPV infections. The best cure is to develop a robust immune system by modifying high-risk sexual behavior and making positive lifestyle changes. Also, keeping up with your regular appointments with your health-care provider will help detect any early changes via your Pap smear.

Questions on Prevention, Vaccination, and Natural Ways To Fight HPV Infections

The answer to the above questions can be clearly understood under the following three subheadings.

Primary Prevention

Primary prevention aims to avoid the development of a disease in a person. This is accomplished in the following ways:

Information, Education, and Communication
Knowledge about the natural history of HPV, transmission, and risk factors are essential. Understanding the difference between high-risk and low-risk types can also be beneficial. In addition, it would be important to keep the public informed about any scientific progress made in order to reduce anxiety and stigmatization (CDC 2000).

Abstinence
The only sure way to prevent HPV is to abstain from all sexual activity. This includes any sexual contact and is not limited to intercourse. Because abstinence is not realistic for most adults, other means of protection must be used to reduce the risk of developing HPV. These may include abstaining from sex when active infected lesions are present, abstaining from unprotected sex, and abstaining from other high-risk sexual behaviors.

Delaying the Age of Sexual Activity
Due to developmental and anatomical reasons, the cervix is more prone to HPV infections and other sexually transmitted infections during the early teen years. Therefore, delaying sexual activity until a later date is advisable.

Being In a Monogamous Relationship
Sexually active adults can greatly reduce their risk of infection by being in a mutually monogamous relationship. But even persons with only one lifetime sex partner can get HPV if their partner has had prior sexual encounters

with other partners. As Dr. Anna Giuliano, professor of Medicine at the H. Lee Moffitt Cancer Center & Research Institute said, "Having sex only once or having only one partner doesn't mean that you are not at risk."

Minimizing the Number of Sexual Partners

Limiting the number of sexual partners that one has in a lifetime can decrease the risk of exposure to HPV. The more sexual partners one has, the greater the exposure and higher the risk of contracting HPV.

Using Barrier Methods

Recent studies have shown that condoms can provide significant (but not total) protection against HPV. Areas that are not covered by the condom can be exposed to the virus. While condoms may not completely prevent sexual transmission of HPV, they can be very helpful in protecting against many other sexually transmitted infections such as HIV, chlamydia, gonorrhea, and herpes. As a precaution, one should always use a barrier method and also learn to use it in the proper manner. Just remember, an ounce of precaution can save you a pound of lifelong trouble and infection.

Avoiding Illicit Drugs and Excessive Alcohol

Avoiding illicit drugs and excessive alcohol can help prevent acquiring HPV because these activities can lead to risky sexual behavior.

Vaccination

Receiving the quadrivalent vaccine *Gardasil* (the only vaccine currently available in the United States) before sexual debut can prevent strains that cause 90 percent of gential warts and 70 percent of cervical cancer. *Cervarix*, which is still not approved in the United States, covers the same two high-risk strains that cause cervical cancer.

Training of Health-Care Professionals

Unfortunately, even health-care professionals lag behind in their understanding of HPV (Kerr et al. 2000). These discussions are time consuming and require competency and knowledge about the link between HPV and cervical and other types of cancer. In addition, health-care providers have to feel comfortable discussing sexually related matters with their patients. Therefore, educating health-care providers is a prerequisite for implementing preventive measures within the community.

> ☞ **The ABCDE of primary prevention of HPV infections are Abstinence, Being monogamous, consistent Condom use, Delaying sexual activity, and Education.**

Secondary Prevention

This step aims to detect the disease in the early stages so that there are adequate opportunities to intervene and prevent progression of the disease. Secondary measures include:

Routine Cervical Screening

Routine cervical screening, such as the Pap test, as suggested by your health-care provider, is still the best way to detect abnormal changes in the cervix.

HPV Testing

This test detects high-risk types of HPV even before there are any conclusive visible changes to the cervical cells. However, The HPV DNA test is not a substitute for regular Pap testing at this time. It also is not intended to screen women under 30 who have normal Pap tests, as most of the infections in this age group clear spontaneously.

Tertiary Prevention

This step is designed to reduce the negative impact of an already established disease by restoring function and reducing further complications. Receiving any difficult diagnosis is hard, but a complication secondary to a STI is even more devastating. An unsightly condition with genital warts or a potential problem with an abnormal Pap smear or a life-threatening condition with cervical cancer can call for minor to sophisticated treatment and from subtle to drastic lifestyle changes. Lifestyle changes are difficult to initiate and even more difficult to maintain. Some of the more straightforward lifestyle changes one has to seriously consider are the following:

Smoking Cessation

Smoking is undeniably bad for you—it was the day you started smoking, it is today, and it will be even worse decades down the road. Along with the numerous documented ill effects caused by smoking, it is also a risk factor for cervical cancer. It weakens the immune system and increases the risk for cancer. The increased risk for cancer starts early, particularly if one is already infected with HPV.

Treatment of Other Sexually Transmitted Diseases

The presence of other sexually transmitted diseases, particularly chlamydia, causes inflammation of the cervix and increases the risk of HPV-induced abnormal changes. Therefore, choose your partner carefully and take precautions.

Treatment of Genital Warts and Abnormal Pap Tests

Genital warts and abnormal Pap tests are managed in several ways as deemed necessary by your health-care professional. It is best to use condoms and dental dams until the active lesions are treated and cleared.

Boosting the Immune System through Holistic Healing

Currently there are no medications to permanently cure or eradicate HPV infections. The closest one can get to fighting HPV infections is by boosting the immune system through holistic healing.

Holistic healing is sadly a widely misunderstood concept. Holistic health does not mean a lifestyle confined to yoga, vegetables, and water. On the contrary, it is the art and science of healing the human body as a whole rather than concentrating on the symptoms alone. It seeks to address the underlying cause for the symptoms by embracing all aspects of the human being—the mind, body, and spirit. The core philosophy of holistic medicine is focusing on patient education and patient participation in the healing process.

Holistic medicine focuses on the belief that a weakened immune system is the root of all ills; the major culprit for the weak immune system is stress. Therefore, holistic health seeks to boost the immune system by adopting various methods and practices that alleviate stress.

When one is under duress for any number of reasons, the body releases high amounts of chemical substances such as adrenaline and cortisol (the flight and fright hormones), which over the long run weaken our body's defenses. Stress reduction lowers the level of these hormones in the body and, thus, helps strengthen the body's immune system and promotes healing. The art of healing comes from a process of self-acceptance, self-embrace, and feeling good about oneself. This can be accomplished in various ways. Some prefer sedentary techniques such as meditation, while others prefer more active practices such as biking, hiking, golf, or jogging. Those who are more visually inclined may benefit from art, walking along the beach and watching a beautiful sunset, while those who are more auditory may prefer to relax with music. In most instances, it is a combination of these methods that people employ to find inner calm. Stress reduction also incorporates physical, nutritional, spiritual, and lifestyle elements. It establishes a relationship between you, your environment, your attitudes, and your beliefs, and gives that much needed emotional relief to strengthen the immune system.

Good nutrition is also key to living a healthy and fulfilling life. As the saying goes, "You are what you eat." Foods such as fruits and vegetables, rich in vitamin C and vitamin E, may reduce the risk of developing cervical cancer. The current recommendations are that everyone should take one multivitamin a day.

Many patients also take herbs on a regular basis to strengthen their immune system. However, more research needs to be done to warrant their use in mainstream practice. Some of the popular herbs used are Ginseng (to adapt to a variety of stressors), Echinacea (to boost the immune system), St. John's Wort (to reduce the accompanying depression), turmeric, and grape seed extract (antioxidants with cancer fighting properties). It should be noted that while herbs have that "natural" cachet, many allopathic medicines include

> ☞ **A healthy lifestyle is the most important factor to prevent HPV infections.**

similar ingredients; therefore people should consider herbs as a form of medication and inform their health-care providers about their intake, especially because some herbs can adversely interact with other medications. To learn more about the official information on dietary supplements, visit the Office of Dietary Supplements at the National Institute of Health's site at http://dietary-supplements.info.nih.gov.

HPV can be a potentially serious and chronic disease that can have a tremendous amount of medical, psychological, and sexual consequences. It can turn your life upside down overnight. One chance encounter is all it takes to be potentially infected by HPV. By seeking authentic information and applying effective coping and preventive skills, one can prevent the spread of HPV. Knowledge and education about HPV infections will help contain the spread of infection. Secrecy and ignorance will not.

KEY FACTS

- The single most important factor to prevent HPV is *education*.
- Knowledge of HPV prevalence is associated with a lower level of stigma, shame, and anxiety.
- Two-thirds to three-fourths of the patients who are diagnosed with HPV experience varying degrees of anxiety, depression, guilt, and fear of rejection.
- A healthy lifestyle is key to preventing and coping with HPV infections.
- Health-care providers should give adequate written information about the emotional, sexual, and medical aspects of HPV disease to their infected patients.

6

The New HPV Vaccines: History, Recommendations, and Limitations

Myth: HPV vaccines will prevent ALL cervical cancers.

Fact: HPV vaccines will protect against only TWO of the cancer-causing strains. Therefore, regular Pap testing is still required for early detection and prevention of all cervical cancers.

Ever since their inception, vaccines have been tough "goods" to sell. In fact, in mid-nineteenth-century England, vaccines were considered to be "filth," and it was punishable by law to inject such substances into humans. Today, most of us would agree that vaccines, inarguably, have been a tremendous boon for mankind. They have dramatically reduced occurrences of debilitating diseases such as polio and smallpox.

Yet, when it comes to the introduction of yet another vaccine to an already large array, both the public and the medical community start off with more doubts than acceptance. Why? In a way, vaccines have become victims of their own success. Due to that phenomenal success, the memory of pandemics from polio, smallpox, and other debilitating illnesses have literally been eroded. This has resulted in attention being diverted from the ravages of diseases to the few potential side effects that the vaccines may have.

People are accustomed to being treated only when they are sick. Vaccines, on the other hand, are administered to perfectly healthy people. Therefore, people see even the slightest of side effects from them as an unacceptable consequence. Scientists have been working for decades to come up with a technology that would make vaccines safer with minimal or no side effects. Their hard work and dedication finally paid off in the development of a breakthrough technology (as we will see later) that was eventually applied to the HPV vaccine.

The Vaccine History—from Bench to Bedside

Timeline

There are fascinating stories behind every scientific discovery, each new story topping the last in how exciting or interesting it is. So, let us take a brief journey back in time to see what twists and turns the HPV vaccine took to get to where it is today.

1842	The first important scientific observation that relates to the future development of the vaccine is made. Domenico Rigoni-Stern, an Italian physician in Verona, notices that among his patients, many prostitutes and married women died of cervical cancer. However, nuns in the nearby convent hardly ever suffered the same fate. Even though he believes that the cancer has something to do with sexual activity, Rigoni-Stern is perplexed and distracted from his original inference by observing that an increasing number of nuns are dying from breast cancer. In his misguided attempt to make a connection, he concludes that the nuns' corsets are dangerously tight.
1901	Dr. Braithwaite, a physician in London, observes that many of his female patients of Jewish descent do not get cervical cancer. He decides the culprit causing cervical cancer is salt and infers that Jewish women are doing well because they have been forgoing the bacon.
1911	The first clue to the link between a virus and certain cancers is established. Dr. F. Peyton Rous, a scientist at the Rockefeller Institute for Medical Research (now Rockefeller University in New York City), shows that sarcoma, a type of cancer occurring in chickens, can be induced in other chickens. He proves his theory by taking an extract from a chicken sarcoma and injecting it into other chickens, causing the other chickens to also get the cancer. Even though this discovery is not met with much enthusiasm at the time, Dr. Rous's work is recognized many years later when he wins the Nobel Prize for Physiology and Medicine in 1966.
1932	The next significant observation is made when Dr. Richard Shope of Rockefeller University is on a hunting trip with his friend. He notices that certain cottontail rabbits grow "giant horns." After returning to work, he tells his friend to send some of these mystical horns to his laboratory. Working with Dr. Rous, he grinds and filters the horns and then injects the filtrate into other rabbits. Interestingly enough, all the rabbits grow horns. These mysterious horns were what we

now know as warts caused by a papillomavirus and were possibly contagious.

1950s   After the formation of Israel, scientists again wonder about the rarity of cervical cancer among Jewish women. They begin to think that rather than the exclusion of bacon from their diets, it might have something to do more with male circumcision (Dunn et al. 1959).

1965   The Epstein-Barr virus, the cause of infectious mononuclosis, is isolated in the lymph node cells of children who suffer from a form of cancer called Burkitt's lymphoma. This becomes the first identified human cancer virus.

1967   Dr. Kamal Abou-Daoud, a physician from the Department of Epidemiology and Biostatistics at the American University of Beirut's School of Public Health in Lebanon, notices that Muslim women with circumcised husbands have rates of cervical cancer just as high as Christian women. In addition, observations of Jewish women from North Africa revealed a significantly higher risk of cervical cancer compared to their counterparts from Israel. Thus, the circumcision theory falls by the wayside.

1970s   Another misleading clue comes to the fore when American physicians find that many women who have cervical cancer also have genital herpes. They erroneously conclude that genital herpes is the cause for cervical cancer (Rawls et al. 1968; Royston & Aurelian 1970).

1980s   Scientists at the National Institutes of Health (NIH) study the bovine (cow) papillomavirus to find out how it alters normal cell behavior and induces tumors. At the same time, reports from Germany start trickling in that a virologist named Harald zur Hausen, together with his colleagues, has isolated the human papillomavirus in nearly 70 percent of cervical cancer biopsies with the help of DNA amplification. This is a "eureka" moment for researchers around the world.

1984   Pharmaceutical companies turn down zur Hausen's request to work on an HPV vaccine. However, his work is quickly followed by a series of studies conducted by the International Agency for Research on Cancer (IARC), which subsequently establishes the causal relationship of HPV to cervical cancer.

1986   In their early work, scientists encounter difficulty in producing enough human papillomaviruses on cultured cells to conduct their experiments. Human warts do not have adequate loads of the virus, so they look for other sources. After many false starts and missteps, the stumbling block is finally overcome when they impregnate bits of foreskin obtained from hospital circumcisions with infected genital wart extract. They then inject this into mice that lack the ability to reject foreign tissue. The cysts that subsequently develop contained enough human papillomaviruses to conduct their experiments.

1990s   There is mounting evidence that HPV causes over 99 percent of cervical cancers, and the race to develop an HPV vaccine is on. However, more scientific challenges remain. Even though sufficient quantities of the human papillomavirus are now available to conduct experiments in the laboratory, scientists strive to develop a technology whereby the vaccine will not contain any viral infectious material.

1994   At this time, there is some talk among HIV/AIDS researchers about using virus-like particles, or VLPs, for making a HIV vaccine (VLPs are made out of the proteins present in the shell that envelopes the viral particles). When these proteins are assembled in a specific way, they serve as the virus's active agent to trigger the body's immune system and produce an antibody to that specific strain of the virus. The VLPs cannot cause infections or cancer because they do not have the viral DNA. This is the first step to developing a vaccine that could save millions of lives around the world.

1994–2006 Scientists devote their time and effort to developing the virus-like particle and taking the technology from bench to bedside. The next roadblock to overcome is to find a way to produce these VLPs in vast quantities for commercialization. Experiments are first carried out in animals (particularly dogs) with the VLP from the corresponding animal papilloma types, and it is found that high levels of antibody are being produced against the corresponding papillomaviruses (Schiller et al. 1996). The quest now begins to develop a HPV VLP that can trigger production of enough antibodies to protect against the human papillomavirus. Work that started on mere hypotheses evolves rapidly into looking for practical solutions to changing the world.

Vaccine Technology

As is the case with any discovery, the road to perfecting the vaccine followed an arduous journey. Developing a vaccine to protect against HPV that did not contain the viral DNA was a daunting task. The virus is difficult to grow on cultured cells, new strains continue to evolve, and clinical trials were difficult to conduct. Eventually, the marvels of genetic engineering came to the rescue.

Vaccines are made in several ways. In order to understand the mechanism by which the HPV vaccine works, we must first understand the workings of our immune systems. The following is a simplified explanation of that.

Our immune system is made up of two parts. The first part is called the humoral immune system. This system produces antibodies that are made by our B lymphocytes. These antibodies circulate in the blood and are available to fight organisms in any location of our bodies, such as the cervical lining. So, when an organism enters a body, the B lymphocytes produce the antibodies, and the antibodies, in turn, reach the intended site to block the organisms *before* they infect the cells. Hence, they prevent the infection from occurring.

This is in stark contrast to the second part of the immune system, which is "cell mediated," or T lymphocyte dependent. Instead of producing antibodies, the T lymphocytes travel to the intended locations themselves. Here, they attack the organism *after* it has entered the cells. They do so by detecting the foreign proteins released from the organism in the infected cells. They then proceed to kill the infected cells, thereby killing the inducing organism in the process.

With this knowledge, let us turn our attention to the vaccine again. Most vaccines that are out on the market today—such as those for measles and mumps—primarily stimulate the humoral immune system to prevent infections; they are preventive (also called prophylactic vaccines). Picture yourself at the doctor's office. When you get a vaccine, it awakens your B lymphocytes to produce antibodies. Then, if the real organism attacks, your body is already well prepared to defend you.

This principle was applied to the HPV vaccine (Stanley et al. 2006). Using technology to manipulate genetic material, scientists discovered that when the major protein, L1, of the outer coat of the virus was assembled in the form of a soccer ball, it looked like the real virus. In that form, the L1 protein, for reasons still unclear, stimulated the B lymphocytes into producing an antibody response that was protective against the targeted HPV types. It is presumed that once these antibodies are produced in the blood, they migrate to the bottommost layer, or basement membrane, of the skin or the mucus lining and work themselves upward toward the topmost layer to wait for the enemy to attack. Therefore, when the real HPV enters the body, the L1 antibodies rapidly bind to the viral proteins and prevent the virus from establishing an infection. The most significant advancement in this method is that the vaccine has no viral infectious DNA whatsoever and, therefore, cannot cause either the infection or the disease.

The medical community often forgets to give gratitude to the unsung heroes in the HPV vaccine quest: the researchers from the National Cancer Institute, the University of Rochester, Georgetown University, and Queensland University in Australia. After 13 years of deliberation, both Merck and GlaxoSmithKline signed royalty agreements with all four institutes so that their original research could be applied to developing and manufacturing the vaccine. Reaching this agreement was in itself a complex human trial of sorts, as numerous pieces of intellectual property rights had to be licensed for appropriate scientific purposes and monetary benefits. It was only after this was accomplished that the actual human trials for the two vaccines could commence.

Clinical Trials: How Was the Vaccine Tested?

Before a drug is introduced to the market for consumer use, it has to go through several phases of medical research, also known as clinical trials. Clinical trials help to determine if a new drug or treatment is safe and effective and how it compares with any existing forms of treatment. Well-conducted clinical trials are the best and safest ways to find new treatments that work.

Scientists enter clinical trials with a great amount of trepidation. It is like getting the report card for years of hard work and labor that went into developing the vaccine. Sometimes they get the result they wish for, while at other times they do not. What may have looked promising in laboratory rats does not always have the same results when tried in humans. What looked like a lifesaver vaccine in the experimental phase may not always translate into decreased number of diseases and deaths in the real world scenario.

As a consumer, there are two aspects of a clinical trial that should be of interest to you: first, how the drug was tested, and, second, how many

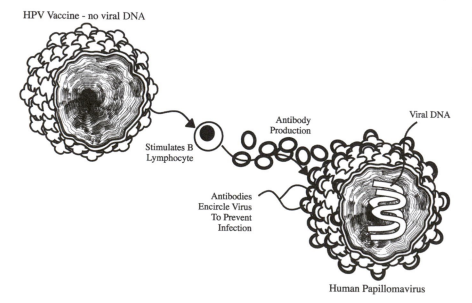

Figure 6.1 Mechanism of Action of HPV Vaccine
Illustrator: Zyamina Gorelik (c) 2008.

subjects it was tested on. For instance, would you accept a vaccine if the researchers said that, in their very extensive and well-documented trials, 33 percent of participants were cured, 33 percent died, and the third subject escaped? Probably not. This old joke reminds us how important it is to assess the type of clinical studies and the number of patients involved in the trials. Obviously, the more studies conducted and the more patients involved from various socioeconomic, cultural, and ethnic backgrounds, the better the results are for consumers.

Clinical trials go through four phases. Phase I marks the earliest trials. They are usually small, and their aim is to study safety, safe dosage range, and side effects of the drug. Once a drug passes phase I (some never do), it goes into phase II trials. These trials involve a larger group of people, usually in the hundreds, to further evaluate the safety and effectiveness of the drug. Once this phase is successfully completed, the drug enters its phase III trials. These trials are usually very large, involving a statistically significant number of patients, usually in the thousands. Their main goal is to study the safety and efficacy of the drug and compare it with other treatments that are available for the same disease. It is based on the success of phase III trials and approval from the Food and Drug Administration (FDA)—the agency that is responsible for the safety regulation for most types of foods and drugs in the United States—that the drug (in this case the vaccine) eventually reaches the market for commercial use.

The next phase, also called phase IV trials or post-marketing trials, commences after the drug is actively prescribed by health-care professionals. The purpose of phase IV trials is to continue to document the safety and side effects of the drug and to detect any rare, long-term, or drug-to-drug interactions, as it is now prescribed to a much larger patient population over a longer period of time.

The two vaccines from Merck and GSK are called the quadrivalent and bivalent vaccines, respectively. The quadrivalent vaccine covers HPV types 6, 11, 16, and 18, hence the name quadrivalent or HPV4. Types 6 and 11 cause 90 percent of anogenital warts; types 16 and 18 cause 70 percent of cervical cancers. The bivalent vaccine, on the other hand, only covers types 16 and 18, hence the name bivalent. It does not cover those types causing genital warts. One can infer that while GSK's focus, (makers of *Cervarix*) was on prevention of cervical cancer, Merck's focus (makers of *Gardasil*) was on broader coverage for the vaccine—the prevention of both cervical cancer and genital warts.

So far, the vaccine trials have each enrolled between 20 and 30 thousand females around the world. One large study called the *FUTURE* (Females United to Unilaterally Reduce Endo/Ectocervical Disease), sponsored by Merck, has two big trials, *FUTURE I* and *FUTURE II*, which are evaluating results at two different end points after the three injection course of the *Gardasil* vaccine or a placebo. An earlier phase of the

FUTURE II study showed that the vaccine was virtually 100 percent effective in preventing infections by the targeted strains for up to 18 months. This study led to the FDA's approval of the Merck's quadrivalent vaccine, *Gardasil,* in 2006.

Large studies are being conducted in the Nordic countries (Norway, Sweden, Finland, Denmark, and Iceland) and in the Latin American country of Costa Rica. Some trials have also enrolled men as a part of their clinical research.

Gardasil was approved in the United States in June 2006. *Cervarix* has recently been approved for use in Australia and the European Union and is expected to receive FDA approval in the United States by late 2008.

Efficacy: Does the Vaccine Really Work?

One of the best methods to assess the effectiveness of a drug is through a randomized, placebo-controlled, double-blind clinical study. Randomized means that there are at least two different groups in the trial and each person is assigned to one group or another at random to receive a different treatment. One group will receive the new treatment being tested, while the other will receive either the standard treatment for the disease or a dummy treatment called a placebo. Those having the standard or placebo treatment are called the control group. A randomized trial that has a control group is called a randomized controlled trial. A placebo is used only if there is no standard treatment available. In the case of the HPV vaccine, there are no other drugs to prevent HPV infections and cervical cancer. Hence, a placebo such as saline water was used. The double-blind trial is the other accepted method to test drugs on humans. A double-blind trial is one in which neither the researchers nor the patients know whether they are getting the drug being tested or the placebo. This method helps to eliminate bias. The computer gives each patient a code number, and the list of patients and their code numbers are kept secret until the end of the trial, unless there is an emergency and the researcher needs to find out immediately what the patient is receiving.

The results of several HPV efficacy trials have now been made available. So far, they have shown that both of the vaccines are nearly 100 percent effective in *preventing* persistent infections and disease caused by the HPV types they cover, provided a person has not been exposed to these specific virus types prior to receiving the vaccine. However, they show that the vaccines are not effective in *treating* HPV infections or disease caused by the vaccine-covered types when they are already present before vaccination. The rest of this subsection is a summary of the efficacy trials for those who are interested.

In order to collect efficacy data in a timely fashion, the vaccine trials depend on easier-to-measure endpoints that, when allowed to progress, would develop into cervical cancer. These include abnormal lesions of the cervix, such as cervical intraepithelial neoplasia (CIN), adenocarcinoma *in situ* (a precancerous lesion that develops in the glandular endocervix and progresses to cancer), vulvar intraepithelial neoplasia (a precancerous lesion of the vulva), and vaginal intraepithelial neoplasia (a precancerous condition of the vagina).

CIN, as we discussed earlier, in turn, is divided into three grades. CIN I is not precancerous and resolves on its own in most cases. About 40 percent of CIN II lesions clear spontaneously. CIN III has the strongest potential to progress to cancer. Hence, CIN II and III, were picked as the end points to determine the effectiveness of the vaccines. These end points are taken as surrogates to cervical cancer, because the cancer itself takes several decades to develop. Besides, using cervical cancer as the end goal of the study would not be an ethical option because such patients would have to be treated much earlier in the disease process in order to prevent them from progressing to the advanced cancer stages.

> ☞ The greatest impact of the vaccine will be in preventing CIN II and CIN III lesions, which, if untreated, may progress to invasive cervical cancer.

The *FUTURE* studies mentioned earlier are further studying the efficacy of *Gardasil*. The first study, the *FUTURE I*, is a randomized, placebo-controlled, double-blind trial conducted on 5,455 girls and women between the ages of 16 and 24. It collects data on any type of external anogenital or cervical lesions, such as warts, and abnormal lesions related to HPV after the vaccine or placebo series. Results from an average three years follow-up has shown that the vaccine was nearly 100 percent effective in preventing genital warts and precancerous lesions in the vulvar, perianal, and cervical regions in women who had not been exposed to HPV types 6, 11, 16, or 18 prior to the study. On the other hand, if a woman had been exposed to any one or more of the HPV stains, either with the vaccine-targeted strains or other stains, it was found that the vaccine was less effective in preventing the various lesions—it reduced vulvar, vaginal, and perianal lesions by only 34 percent regardless of the HPV types, and reduced the occurrence of cervical lesions by 20 percent regardless of HPV types.

The second study, *FUTURE II*, which is also a randomized, placebo-controlled, double-blind trial, is being conducted on 12,157 girls and women aged 15–26 from 90 study areas in 13 countries. Results from an average three years follow-up showed that the vaccine was 98–100 percent effective in preventing high-grade precancerous lesions (CIN II or CIN III) after receiving the vaccine series. However, the vaccine was only 44 percent effective in the group of women who were included regardless of their prior exposure to any HPV types.

Therefore, both studies have shown that the vaccine was most effective in preventing and not treating HPV infections, and it worked best when administered before sexual debut.

Similar results have been seen with *Cervarix,* confirming that it is also a prophylactic (preventive) vaccine and not a therapeutic (for treatment) vaccine. Interim data from phase III trials with *Cervarix* have now been released and show that the vaccine is almost 100 percent effective in preventing significant cervical lesions with the vaccine targeted strains of 16 and 18. Studies also contained data to show that the vaccine offers cross-protection against other HPV types—particularly 45 and 31, which are the third and fourth most common causes of cervical cancer. A press release by GSK in March 2008 announced that *Cervarix* was 78 percent effective against HPV type 45 and 60 percent effective against HPV type 31. *Cervarix* also seems to lend coverage against HPV type 52, which is also one of the cancer-causing types. Globally, the most oncogenic types are HPV 16, which accounts for 53 percent of all cervical cancers, followed by HPV 18 with 17.2 percent, HPV 45 with 6.7 percent, and HPV 31 with 2.9 percent (Adams et al. 2007). Due to this added benefit from its broader range of coverage, *Cervarix* may be effective against 80 percent of cervical cancers.

Trials are also being conducted to look at the effectiveness of *Gardasil* on anogenital lesions. Results have shown that the vaccine significantly reduces the incidence of anogenital diseases. This could also indicate that the vaccine may provide protection against other diseases caused by HPV 6, 11, 16, and 18. Recent data also shows that *Gardasil* may also confer a modicum of cross-protection against 10 additional (31, 33, 35, 39, 45, 51, 52, 56, 58, and 59) cancer-causing types of HPV strains not targeted by the vaccine (Roehr 2007).

One might ask, how do we already know that the vaccines are really effective if cervical cancer takes several years to develop? To be honest, no one will know the real answer for decades. The final efficacy of the vaccines in cancer prevention will require long-term follow-ups of a large group of vaccinated women. If girls who are 11 and 12 years old and not sexually active are getting the vaccines now, given the relatively long induction phase between exposure to the HPV cancer-causing strains and the development of cancer, it will take at least another 25–40 years to know if they were protected by the vaccine.

The vaccine has been approved in 9–15-year-old girls based on the clinical results seen in women between the ages of 16 and 24 who are enrolled in the current study.

☞ Both *Gardasil* and *Cervarix* are preventive vaccines and not therapeutic vaccines.

Such a study is called an immunology bridging study. In such a study, blood antibody levels (also called antibody titers, which are currently used only for research purposes in the case of HPV) were measured in the 9- to 15-year olds one month after the vaccine series. It was found that the vaccine-induced responses in this age group were substantially higher than the vaccine-induced response observed in 16–24-year-old women, the age group in which 98–100 percent preventive efficacy has been demonstrated. It was thus derived that the administration of the HPV vaccine to young adolescents in the 9–15-year-old group should induce similar if not better protective efficacy, as their blood antibody titers were even higher. It is based on such a modeling study that the vaccines have been approved for boys, too, in parts of the European Union and Australia. Clinical studies are currently in progress in boys and men in the United States, and the results should be available within the next couple of years.

Duration of Immunity: How Long Are the Vaccines Good?

The duration of vaccine protection will not be known until long-term follow-ups are completed. However, from what we know at this time from the efficacy studies, *Gardasil* has shown significant antibody protection against HPV types 6, 11, 16, and 18 for *at least* five years (Villa et al. 2006).

The rest of this chapter will focus predominantly on the quadrivalent vaccine, *Gardasil,* as it is the only one approved by the FDA in the United States so far. Information about the bivalent vaccine will also be discussed throughout the chapter wherever available.

VACCINE DETAILS

Current Recommendations

The current recommendations by the Advisory Committee on Immunization Practices (ACIP)—an arm of the Centers for Disease Control and Prevention (CDC), the American Association of Family Practice

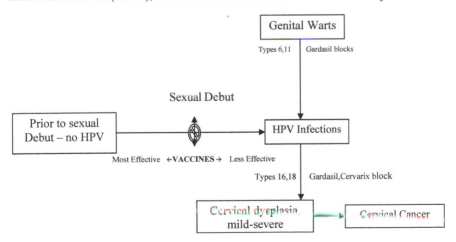

Figure 6.2 Where the HPV Vaccines Work

(AAFP), and the American Association of Pediatrics (AAP)—for the quadrivalent vaccine are as follows:

- Routine vaccination of females 11–12 years of age with three doses of quadrivalent HPV vaccine.
- The vaccination series can be started as young as nine years of age (at the parent's and physician's discretion).
- The vaccination is also recommended for females between the ages of 13 and 26 years who have not been previously immunized or have not completed the whole series.

Rationale behind the Current Recommendation

As the vaccine is for prevention and not for treatment of HPV infections, it is best to vaccinate girls before they become sexually active (refer to Figure 6.2). This recommendation was based on the following statistics from the National Survey of Family Growth (NSFG; an agency that collects information on American teen sexual behavior) in 2005:

- Thirteen percent of high school students have had sexual experience by age 15.
- Forty-three percent of females become sexually active by age 17.
- Seventy percent of females become sexually active by age 19.
- Seventy percent of 13–21-year olds have had evidence of HPV infections within five to seven years of onset of sexual intercourse.

In adolescence, the ability to immunize is limited because many do not receive annual health exams. Therefore, from a public health perspective, routine vaccination at 11–12 years of age is the best way to attain wide-scale immunization.

Indications—What Is the Vaccine Used For?

Gardasil is currently indicated to prevent the following diseases:

- Cervical cancer
- Abnormal and precancerous cervical lesions
- Abnormal and precancerous vaginal lesions
- Abnormal and precancerous vulvar lesions
- Genital warts

Dose Schedule

The vaccine is administered per the following schedule:

First dose—At elected date
Second dose—2 months after the first dose
Third dose—6 months after the first dose

Alternate Schedules

First dose—Minimum age: nine years old
Second dose—Minimum interval: 4 weeks after first dose
Third dose—Minimum interval: 12 weeks after second dose

Interrupted Vaccine Schedules

Vaccine schedules sometimes get interrupted for various reasons. This is particularly true on college campuses where students might leave for a whole semester to study abroad and miss the deadline to get the vaccines on a scheduled basis.

If the *Gardasil* vaccine schedule is interrupted, the vaccine series *does not need* to be restarted. If the schedule is interrupted after the first dose, the second dose should be given as soon as possible. The third dose can be given 12 weeks after the second dose. If that time interval is missed, the third dose should be administered as soon as possible.

Catch-up Vaccination of Females Aged 13–26 Years

Even though the vaccination is recommended for 11–12-year-old girls, the CDC also recommends that the vaccine be offered to older girls and young women on the premise that even if they have been exposed to HPV, they may not have been exposed to all the strains covered by the vaccine.

Dosage and Administration

0.5 ml of the vaccine is administered intramuscularly in the deltoid muscle of the arm.

Simultaneous Administration with Other Vaccines

The vaccine can be administered with other age-appropriate vaccines such as tetanus, diphtheria, meningococcal, and hepatitis B. At this time, data is only available with the simultaneous administration of the hepatitis B vaccine. The HPV vaccine should not be mixed in a syringe with any other vaccines; each vaccine should be administered with a separate needle and syringe at different anatomic sites.

Cancer Screening among Vaccinated Females: Should Vaccinated Women Who Are Sexually Active Still Get Pap Tests?

The vaccine does not cover all types of cancer-causing HPV. Hence, Pap tests should be continued in all vaccinated women, per ACS guidelines.

HPV Testing: Should HPV Testing Be Done before Receiving the Vaccine Series?

HPV testing is not recommended before the vaccination series. The test does not detect past infections, nor does it distinguish among various oncogenic HPV types. In addition, as the vaccine covers more than one HPV type, it could still be beneficial even if a person has already been exposed to one or more types.

Special Situations among Vaccine-eligible Females

Vaccination of Sexually Active Women

Results from *FUTURE I* and *FUTURE II* studies show that sexually active women may expect to benefit from the vaccine, but not as much as those who have not been exposed to the covered HPV types—44 versus 98 percent. The CDC recommends the vaccine up to 26 years of age.

Vaccination of Older Women

Divorced women, remarried women, and older women who are single and sexually active may continue to be exposed to HPV throughout their lives. Therefore, *Cervarix* has now been approved in women up to age 45 in countries outside the United States. The drug company is currently seeking approval for women up to the age of 55. *Gardasil* is approved for women until the age of 26, and Merck is seeking approval for *Gardasil* in older women up to the age of 45 as well.

Vaccination of Women with Abnormal Pap Smears

Women who have a low-grade abnormality on their Pap smears may not be infected with all the oncogenic HPV types covered by the vaccine. Therefore, they may be viable candidates for the vaccine. However, as the severity of the abnormality increases, their chances of being infected by HPV types 16 and 18 also go up proportionately, and therefore, the benefit of the vaccine decreases. *Gardasil* also covers types 6 and 11, which can give protection against 90 percent of genital warts, if a woman has not already been exposed to those types. Again, it should be noted that HPV is a viral infection with no cure, and the vaccine is prophylactic and only prevents infection prior to being exposed to the virus. It is best to consult your health-care professional for your individual needs.

Vaccination during Pregnancy

Vaccination is not recommended during pregnancy, as data on this group is limited. If the woman is found to be pregnant after initiation of the series, it is best to postpone the remainder of the vaccines until after childbirth. So far there is limited data on the adverse effects of *Gardasil* on pregnancy outcomes or fetal abnormalities. In addition, as of now, there is *no* indication to terminate the pregnancy if the vaccine is inadvertently administered to a woman who is pregnant. However, all women who receive the vaccine during pregnancy should notify the *Gardasil* pregnancy registry by dialing 1-800-986-8999. This registry collects information to monitor the effects of the vaccine on pregnancies. Individual patient information is kept confidential.

Vaccination in Women with Genital Warts

Genital warts are usually caused by HPV types 6 and 11. But, women with genital warts may not be carriers of types 16 and 18. Hence, in such women, vaccination with *Gardasil* is recommended with the caveat that the vaccines will not have any effect on the existing infections or genital warts.

Vaccination in Lactating Women

Women who are breastfeeding their babies can receive the vaccine.

Vaccination in Women with a Weakened Immune System

As the vaccine has no infectious material, it can be given to women whose immune system has been weakened due to medication such as steroids or from diseases that compromise the immune system such as HIV/AIDS. It is to be noted that the immune response and the effectiveness of the vaccine may be blunted.

Groups for Whom the Vaccine Is Not Licensed

Age Limits

Gardasil is not recommended for females aged less than nine years or older than 26 years. *Cervarix* is not recommended for females aged less than 10 years or older than 45 years.

Men

The vaccines have not been licensed for use in men in the United States at this time. Currently there is positive data available on the antibody levels and safety in males; whether these parameters translate into effectiveness is still not known. Efficacy studies in males are underway in the United States.

Side Effects, Precautions, and Contraindications

All adverse events to a vaccine that are clinically significant are customarily reported by the clinic or the physician's office to a branch of the U.S. Department of Health Services: the Vaccine Adverse Event Reporting

System (VAERS). VAERS collects data on all potential associations between vaccines and adverse effects, whether it is coincidental or truly caused by the vaccine. VAERS can be reached at 1-888-822-7967. Electronic forms for reporting are also available at https://secure.vaers.org/ VaersDataEntryintro.htm to promote prompt reporting and better safety data.

Most Commonly Reported Side Effects

The most commonly reported side effects are

- Pain at the injection site (about 8 in 10 people).
- Redness or swelling at the site of injection (about 1 in 4 people).
- Mild fever (100 degrees Fahrenheit) or less (about 1 in 10 people).
- Fainting or passing out spells (also known as syncope; about 1 in 10 people).
- Nausea (about 4 in 100 people).
- Dizziness (about 3 in 100 people).

Syncope (a condition where there is temporary loss of conciousness with spontaneous recovery) can occur after any vaccination and is a common occurrence among adolescents between 10 and 18 years of age. According to the CDC, about 50 percent of adolescents and young adults experience at least one episode of syncope at some point. The most common reasons for their occurrences in this age group are fear of needles and erratic eating patterns. Fortunately, minor side effects are short-lived and resolve on their own.

So far, no specific side effects have been reported in people with chronic diseases such as diabetes, seizures, or attention deficit syndromes. In addition, no drug interactions have been reported with other medications.

Serious Side Effects

VAERS defines serious adverse effects as those that involve a life-threatening illness, hospitalization, death or disability, or any other medically important condition after administration of a vaccine. So far, VAERS's report on *Gardasil* is as follows:

As of April 30, 2008, VAERS received a total of 5,070 reports related to the HPV vaccine. Of these, 95 percent were classified as non-serious. So far, adverse reactions to *Gardasil* have been lower than average. The five most common serious adverse reactions associated with the use of *Gardasil* were vomiting, syncope, fever, nausea, and headache.

Forty-two percent of serious adverse events occurred on the day of vaccination or within 24–48 hours. The data also showed that there were 31 reports of Guillain-Barre syndrome (GBS). GBS is a disorder in which the body's immune system affects part of the nervous system causing weakness and tingling of extremities. Most patients recover from it completely. Of the 31 cases reported, six received Gardasil alone, out of which only two met the case definition of GBS. Symptoms occurred within six weeks of vaccination in both cases. Five involved co-administration of *Menactra* (the meningitis vaccine) and *Gardasil*. One received *Gardasil, Menactra,* and the Hepatitis A vaccine, and one received *Gardasil* and Pneumococcal Polysaccharide Vaccine given within 30 days of one another. According to the CDC, GBS occus at a rate of 1–2 per 100,000 persons per year in young adults. Therefore, these cases may be coincidental and not causal findings. The other reports are currently being investigated.

As of April 30, 2008, VAERS reported 15 deaths after the administration of the *Gardasil* vaccine. Only 10 reports contained the necessary information needed for further analysis. Of these, most deaths were associated with known causes in the respective age groups, and did not seem to be causally related to vaccination. For example, two died from the complications of influenza and happened to have received the HPV vaccine. Another two involved a blood clot, one in the lung and one in the leg. Both these patients were taking birth control pills—fatal blood clots are a rare side effect of this medication. The occurrence of these clots was consistent with that experienced when taking birth control pills alone. The CDC, however, is continuing to monitor a variety of safety outcomes including Guillian-Barre syndrome, seizure, syncope, stroke, and blood clots.

In summary, considering that over 12 million doses of the vaccine have been distributed to date, the adverse effects remain relatively rare. At this time, there is no way to know how many doses have been actually administered, because the United States does not maintain a national registry for immunization.

Gardasil is also covered under the National Vaccine Injury Compensation Program since February 1, 2007. No claims alleging injuries had been filed as of June 7, 2007. For further updates, please visit http://www.cdc.gov/vaccines/vpd-vac/hpv/downloads/hpv-gardasil-gbs.pdf.

Precautions

Syncope
As mentioned earlier, syncope is one of the most common side effects after vaccination. Precaution should be taken in those who have had a passing-out spell with prior vaccinations. It is therefore best for patients to be observed in the clinic or doctor's office for a minimum of 15 minutes after the vaccination.

Acute Illnesses
Low grade fever, cough, diarrhea, and other mild illnesses are not contraindications to the vaccination. However, if a person has moderate to severe illness, it is best to postpone the vaccination.

Contraindications (Who Should Not Receive the Vaccine)

Allergy to Vaccine Components
The vaccine should not be given to anyone who is hypersensitive to any of the vaccine components, such as yeast. *Gardasil* is grown on yeast and therefore should not be administered to anyone with severe allergic reaction to yeast. *Cervarix* is not grown on yeast.

HPV Vaccines: Overview

Table 6.1 summarizes many of the salient points discussed thus far in this chapter. The information provided is a quick guide and primer for the many queries one may have about the vaccines at any given time.

Public Implications of the Vaccine

Cost and Reimbursement

The vaccine, despite its new technology, does not come cheap to consumers. In fact, covering the cost of the vaccine series has some stakeholders bristling at the notion of school requirements, even if they believe that the vaccine had some definitive merits. The average price is $120 per dose plus an administration fee for each vaccine. The vaccine is available to eligible 9- to 18-year olds through the "Vaccines for Children Program" and via Medicaid to 19- to 21-year olds.

Vaccine for Children Program (VFC)

Every state has a VFC to provide recommended childhood vaccines free to eligible children. There is no out-of-pocket expense for the vaccine to either the parents or the health-care provider, but providers may charge a nominal fee to cover the cost of administering the vaccine.

If a patient cannot afford to pay the provider's fees, the law requires that the provider still administer the vaccine to the patient. Parents of children enrolled in Medicaid programs should not be charged an administrative fee. To be reimbursed, the provider should bill the state Medicaid program. Detailed information about the VFC program is available on the CDC Web site (http://cdc.gov/). Once you are on the CDC Web site, enter "VFC" to learn more about the Vaccines for Children program.

Children Who Are Eligible for the VFC Vaccine
Children are eligible for VFC vaccines if they are 18 years of age or younger and meet one of the following criteria:

- Are eligible for Medicaid;
- Have no health insurance;

Table 6.1 Overview of HPV Vaccines

Category	Quadrivalent (*Gardasil*) (Merck)	Bivalent (*Cervarix*) (GlaxoSmithKline).
Vaccine type	Preventive—does not treat HPV infections.	Same.
HPV types included	6, 11, 16, and 18 VLPs Quadrivalent (four types).	16 and 18 VLPs Bivalent (covers two types)
Clinical trials	17,800 women (ages 16–26), 3,800 women (ages 18–25), 3,700 men (ages 16—24). Trials continue through 2008. Tested around the world. The vaccine has been tested on a little over 1,000 girls between the ages of 9 and 15.	18,000 women (ages 15 to 25), 12,000 women (ages 18 to 25). Trials continue through 2010.
Vaccine component	Viral capsid L1 protein.	Same.
Infectivity	Does not have any HPV DNA particle. Hence, noninfectious and does not cause cancer.	Same.
Adjuvant (helper chemical or an immune boosting agent that helps to enhance the effect of a vaccine without having any antigenic effects of its own)	Contains amorphous aluminium hydroxyphosphate sulfate. This is the only adjuvant that is approved by the FDA for use in vaccines.	Contains a proprietary innovative adjuvant AS04 (aluminium hydroxide + monophosphoryl lipid A). The addition of the bacterial lipid supposedly confers a stronger, higher, and longer antibody levels compared to any other adjuvant.
Thiomerosal or mercury content in vaccine	None.	None.

Culture that it is grown in	Yeast.	Baculovirus (virus that infects insects).
Efficacy in preventing cervical abnormality and cervical cancer	98%–100% effective against 70% of all cervical cancers. Additional cross-protection may exist.	Nearly 100% effective against 80% of all cervical cancers due to cross-protection.
Efficacy in preventing genital warts	Almost 100% effective against 90% of genital warts.	No protection against genital warts.
Cross-protection (decreased risk of infection from one or more strains that are not targeted by the vaccines)	Newer studies showing some evidence of cross-protection against 10 additional strains.	Types 45, 31, and 52; has 78% protection against type 45 and 60% protection against type 31. Types 45 and 31 are the third and fourth most common cervical cancer-causing viruses.
Duration of protection	At least up to 5 years at the present time.	At least up to 5 years at the present time.
Dosage schedule	0, 2, and 6 months.	Not yet approved in the United States.
Eligible age	Females 9–26 years	Not yet approved in the United States.
Optimum time to vaccinate	Before onset of sexual activity. Current recommendations are to vaccinate 11–12-year-old girls.	Before onset of sexual activity. Currently not available in the United States.
Adverse effects	Pain at injection site, syncope, dizziness, nausea.	Too early to report—recently introduced into the Australian and European markets.
Contraindications	Hypersensitivity to any of the vaccine components or yeast.	Hypersensitivity to any of the vaccine components.

Concurrent illness	Can be administered in the presence of other acute illnesses such as a common cold or diarrhea.	No recommendations available for the U.S. market.
Administration in immunocompromised patients	The vaccine can be administered.	No recommendations available for the U.S. market.
Cervical screening	Routine screening should continue after vaccination.	Routine screening should continue after vaccination.
Pregnancy and breast feeding	Should not be administered to pregnant women but can be given to lactating women.	Recommendations not yet available for the U.S. market.

- Are Native American or Alaskan Native; or
- Have health insurance, but it does not cover immunizations. In these cases, these children must go to a Federally Qualified Health Center (FQHC) or Rural Health Clinic (RHC) for immunizations.

Providers of the Free Vaccine Program

The free vaccine can be obtained from any organization or institution enrolled as a provider in the VFC Program. VFC program providers can include:

- Private doctors' offices
- Private clinics
- Hospitals
- Public health clinics
- Community health clinics
- Certain schools in some states

State Children's Health Insurance Program (SCHIP)

Those states that have a SCHIP program that operates separately from the Medicaid program will cover ACIP approved vaccines for their beneficiaries.

Private Insurance Companies

Private Insurance companies who cover other ACIP recommended vaccines will now cover the HPV vaccine. However, there could be some geographical variations.

Merck Vaccine Patient Assistance Program

Merck has also established the Merck Vaccine Patient Assistance Program to offer the vaccine to eligible adults who are uninsured. For more information, contact (800) 293-3881.

New Hampshire has implemented a free voluntary HPV vaccine program for girls 18 and younger. This program is jointly funded by the federal government and private insurers and has been a very successful program.

Health Benefits of the Vaccine

Several studies have been conducted to evaluate the impact of the HPV vaccine. One cost-benefit analysis model suggested that vaccination of girls against high-risk HPV subtypes would be cost-effective if administered under certain parameters: if all 12-year-old girls currently living in the United States were vaccinated, their lifetime risk of cervical cancer could be reduced by 20–66 percent depending on the duration of immunity and the effectiveness of the vaccine (Sanders & Taira 2003; Goldie et al. 2004).

Current obstacles to public health benefits include poor access to the general public, particularly the uninsured, the underinsured, and women in the low socioeconomic strata.

Future Promise

More research is underway to develop second- and third-generation vaccines that can not only prevent but also treat and cover a broader range of oncogenic strains of HPV. Therapeutic vaccines offer a much greater promise than prophylactic vaccines, as they are likely to treat the clinical manifestations of the virus such as warts, precancerous lesions and perhaps even cervical cancer. Though they sound practical in concept, the technology to develop them is much more challenging than that to produce preventive vaccines. Other research in vaccine technology includes alternate routes of administration such as skin patches, intranasal sprays, and development of methods to enhance and sustain a strong and robust immune response.

> ☞ **The success rate of the vaccination program will be greatest when preadolescents and adolescents who are at highest risk of cervical cancer have access to the vaccine.**

CONCLUSION

HPV vaccines look promising. The vaccines appear to be very effective against those strains that are predominantly responsible for the majority of cervical cancers. If guidelines to time of administration and doses are followed, there can be a considerable reduction in the disease incidence and death associated with HPV-related diseases. At this time, the success rate in preventing cervical cancer with the current vaccines will be of greatest magnitude to those preadolescents and adolescents who are unlikely to undergo regular Pap smears either due to poor awareness or poor access to health care, or a combination of both.

In the future, the vaccines may also be found to protect against many types of vulvar, vaginal, anal, penile, and oral cancers caused by HPV types.

The vaccines, however, have some limitations. First of all, not all cervical cancers are caused by HPV 16 or HPV 18. Second, patients have to be vaccinated before being exposed or infected by the virus in order for the vaccine to be fully effective. Finally, the long-term side effects and their effectiveness in preventing cervical cancer will not be realized for decades. Women will still need to take precautions such as using condoms and other barrier methods. In addition, they will still need their regular cervical cancer screening from their clinicians.

KEY FACTS

- There are two HPV vaccines now available in the world markets. Only one, *Gardasil*, has so far been approved for use in the United States. The second vaccine, *Cervarix*, is awaiting FDA approval and may be available in late 2008.
- Both *Gardasil* and *Cervarix* are preventive vaccines. They do not treat for active HPV infections or HPV-related diseases.
- Due to the preventive nature of the vaccines, it is best to vaccinate girls before they come in contact with HPV.
- The vaccine is not approved for boys or men in the United States at this time.
- The vaccines do not contain any infectious part of HPV and, therefore, cannot cause cancer.
- Three doses of the vaccine are required to develop adequate immunity. It is not known at this time if booster shots will be required in the future.
- The vaccines will not prevent all types of cervical cancers. Therefore, regular cervical cancer screenings such as Pap tests are still required.
- HPV vaccines will not prevent other STIs such as herpes or gonorrhea. Sexually active people should therefore take the routine and customary steps to reduce exposure to STIs.

7

HPV Vaccines for Males: The Unsolved Half of the Equation

Myth: Men do not suffer from any HPV-related cancers.

Fact: HPV causes nearly as many cancers in men as it does cervical cancer in women. Men can also transmit the virus to women and increase their risk of cervical cancer—a real threat that cannot be ignored.

People around the world have heard of María Eva Duarte de Perón, the famous first lady of Argentina from 1946 to 1952 who was better known by her nickname Evita. Even though she was well known in her time as a humanitarian, she was made even more famous after her death by the hugely popular Broadway musical and subsequent 1996 Hollywood movie, also titled "Evita." She was the second wife of President Juan Perón of Argentina. When she fell ill, Eva's husband and her doctors went to great lengths to keep her illness a secret for political reasons. Many people know that, ultimately, Eva Perón died from her illness; what they do not know is that this illness was cervical cancer.

In the mid-twentieth century, very little was known about the link between Eva's cervical cancer and the sexually transmitted virus HPV. Today, many scientists believe that she probably caught HPV from her husband, whose first wife also died of cervical cancer. This celebrity story sheds light on the potentially real threat of men passing this silent virus to their female partners, and, subsequently, causing the women to develop life-threatening cervical cancer (Bosch et al. 1996).

Even though cervical cancer is the most widely recognized disease caused by HPV, the virus does not just present a risk in women. HPV can cause significant health risks in men too. HPV is responsible for causing genital warts and anal, penile, mouth, and throat cancers in men.

In addition, it should not be forgotten that HPV is spread to women through sexual contact with men in the majority of cases. Therefore, an understanding of HPV infections in men is critical in reducing the risk of transmission to women.

So, if men are at such risk and play such an integral role in the transmission of HPV, why are they not being targeted equally by HPV prevention programs such as the "ONE LESS" campaign for *Gardasil*? The answer might lie in the sheer lack of information. While a wealth of information about HPV in women is available, research on the virus in men has so far only scratched the surface. Far more research has been done on HPV in women because, traditionally, infections have been considered less serious in men. Lately, bits and pieces of information about HPV in men have been brought to the fore from various studies in different settings, and these studies should eventually fill the information gaps regarding HPV infections in men.

The questions regarding HPV infections in men are numerous. Experts have long wondered how HPV infections are acquired and transmitted among men, how frequently men transmit infections to women, and whether it is safe for a man to continue to have sexual contact with male or female partners if he is infected. With the advent of cervical cancer vaccinations, experts have also asked if vaccinating men would help reduce the incidence of cervical cancer in women, and, even if the answer to this question were yes, if men would take the incentive to get the vaccine to protect their future female sexual partners. While most of these questions still do not have concrete answers, it is important to first examine what we already know about HPV infections in men in order to understand how the vaccines, when approved for men, might benefit the population at large.

HPV INFECTIONS IN MEN—PREVALENCE RATES

The overall prevalence rate of HPV infections (the total number of persons carrying HPV at any given time) among sexually active men is high. In order to better understand the nature of HPV infections in men, a group of scientists and physicians from the CDC looked at 40 different publications on the prevalence of HPV infections in the male population (Dunne et al. 2006). Their conclusion was that more than half of American men will get HPV infections at some point in their lives.

Prevalence rates in men range anywhere from 20 to 72.9 percent based on factors such as age, race or ethnicity, circumcision status, tobacco smoking, and sexual orientation. It has further been shown that the rate of infection in men, when compared to women, is more constant among men in all age groups. In women, the highest rates of infection are seen in their twenties, with rates then decreasing in their thirties and surging again in their forties and fifties, either due to reactivation of dormant infections or reinfection from men.

As very few scientific studies exist between the association of men and HPV-associated diseases, numerous myths, theories, and conjectures about HPV and men abound. The research conducted so far has helped us better understand the prevalence of HPV in the different categories of men.

College-aged Men

A study conducted at the University of Washington among 240 hetero-sexually active men between the ages of 18 and 20 showed that nearly 66 percent of these men developed HPV within two years of initiating sexual activity. One of the most commonly detected types was HPV 16, the type that causes more than 50 percent of cervical cancers. HPV types were found in various locations on the male genitals, including the penile shaft, the tip of the penis (also called the glans penis), and the scrotum. Among the factors associated with increased risk were young age, unprotected sex, higher number of sex partners, higher frequency of sexual intercourse, and cigarette smoking.

Men Who Have Sex with Men (MSM)—Gay and Bisexual Men

Studies estimate that the prevalence of HPV in the anal canals of MSM who are HIV negative and have receptive anal sex ranges anywhere from 60 to 75 percent, and the prevalence of HPV in HIV-positive MSM ranges from 80 to 100 percent depending on how compromised their immune systems are. This high prevalence is consistent among all age groups and is attributed to the sexual practices of MSM, who tend to have more new sexual partners after the age of 30 than do women over the age of 30. In addition, 23 percent of HIV-negative and 61 percent of HIV-positive men are infected with multiple HPV types, including high-risk types. HIV-positive men are four to five times more likely to contract HPV infections than HIV-negative men. They are also more prone to infections with multiple HPV types. Several studies have suggested that having multiple types of HPV increases the risk of progression to anal cancer. Nearly 90 percent of anal cancers are HPV positive and are caused mostly by HPV type 16. However, as is the case with women, most men with a robust immune system are able to clear the infection without any development of disease or cancer.

Men Using Condoms

The prevalence of low-risk and high-risk types of HPV among men who use condoms correctly and consistently is low. Condom labeling for STIs including HPV have been the center of a political debate for years. As HPV can be spread by skin-to-skin contact, conservative groups and abstinence-only advocates proclaim that condoms provide little protection from HPV.

In order to understand the relationship between consistent and correct condom use and HPV prevalence and transmission, a 4-1/2-year long study was conducted by the University of Washington among 82 sexually active female students. The women who participated in this study had either initiated sexual intercourse with a new male partner during the study or within two weeks before it began. Electronic diaries were used, so that women would be more truthful about their condom use than if they were confronted face to face. It was found that women whose partners used condoms 100 percent of the time during intercourse for eight months since program inception were 70 percent less likely to acquire new infections than women whose partners used condoms less than 5 percent of the time. Women who used condoms more than half the time were also 50 percent less likely to have HPV infections that those who rarely or never used them. These results remained true even after adjusting for a very critical variable—number of sexual partners. Furthermore, the study suggested that consistent condom use reduced the risk of acquiring both low-risk and high-risk types of HPV, which could have a significant impact in reducing the incidence of diseases such as genital warts and HPV-related cancers. This study, even though it was small, was specifically designed to explore the relationship between frequency of condom use and HPV infections. In addition, information from participants was collected every two weeks as opposed to months or years later as previous studies had done. This, along with the use of computer-based diaries, yielded a more truthful reporting of a sensitive behavior (Winer et al. 2006).

In addition, two earlier studies done in the Netherlands in 2003 suggested that consistent use of condoms could speed the clearance of the HPV-related lesions on the cervix and on the penis and shorten the time needed to clear HPV infections. These two studies, though not designed to show if condoms reduced the risk of transmission of HPV, nevertheless added helpful evidence that condoms facilitated the regression of HPV-related diseases in those who used them consistently and correctly.

☞ **Consistent condom use reduces HPV transmission by 70 percent.**

All of the above findings may have the potential to change the tide for condom use to minimize the spread of HPV infections.

Circumcised Men

The role of circumcision in the prevention of diseases in men has been a subject of intense controversy. In the United States, an estimated 80 percent of newborn males were circumcised in the 1970s. However, the rates subsequently declined after the American Academy of Pediatrics issued a policy stating that there was no sufficient evidence to recommend newborn circumcision. But recently, there is mounting evidence to show that the prevalence of both high-risk and low-risk HPV types among circumcised men is significantly lower, in the range of 20 to 70 percent reduction when compared to uncircumcised men. This reduction in prevalence gives a biologically plausible explanation for the reduced risk of genital HPV infections in men and a concomitant reduced risk of cervical cancer in women, particularly in those with high-risk sexual partners (Castellsagué et al. 2002).

During the process of circumcision, the prepuce, or the part of the foreskin covering the tip of the penis, is removed. This minimizes the mini-abrasions and the total surface area through which HPV can enter the skin. Circumcision also causes the skin of the tip of the penis to get thicker and provide a protective shield against HPV. In addition, circumcision makes it easier to maintain good penile hygiene by eliminating the collection of smegma, a cheese-like secretion that accumulates under the foreskin that is conducive to harboring HPV. Circumcision also minimizes the risk of other sexually transmitted infections such as chlamydia, which can act as a cofactor in the acquisition of HPV infections.

From a public health standpoint it should be pointed out that circumcision, by itself, does not protect against cervical cancer. Rather, it protects against cervical cancer by reducing the incidence of HPV infections.

Socioeconomics and Ethnic Minorities

Prevalence rates are higher among ethnic minorities and the economically disadvantaged. HPV prevalence is highest among African American and Hispanic men from the South and in white men from the Appalachian region where tobacco smoking is high, circumcision rates are low, and penile hygiene is poor—all risk factors for HPV infections.

HPV Associated Conditions in Men: From Head and Neck to Anal Diseases

In most cases, HPV does not produce any symptoms in men, as it tends to resolve by itself. In the cases when symptoms do appear, the changes are often minor and hardly noticeable. HPV infections in men, much like in women, are passed through genital contact and sex. HPV gains access through tiny abrasions in the skin of the base of the penis, penile shaft, scrotum, anus, and, areas surrounding it. HPV can cause serious diseases in men such as anal, penile, mouth, and throat cancers.

The statistics in Table 7.1 strongly highlight the association between HPV and its related cancers in men. When taking a closer look, it is very evident that these statistics run almost parallel to the statistics of cervical cancer cases that occur in women in the United States annually. This observation alone should be convincing enough to change the

Table 7.1 Approximate Number of New Cases of HPV-related Diseases in Males in the United States Annually

Disease	Number of new cases per year	% with detectable HPV	Number of new HPV-related cases
Recurrent respiratory papillamatosis	approximately 3,300	100%	all 3,300/year
Genital warts	approximately 500,000	100%	all 500,000 cases/year
Cancer of mouth and throat	25,830	26.9 %	6,948/year
Anal cancers	1,910	90%	1,719/year
Penile cancers	1,530	50%	765/year
Total number of new HPV-related cancers	...	...	9,432/year

Source: Based on information from the American Cancer Society.

general perception that only women are at risk from HPV. The following section is an overview of the HPV-related diseases possible in men.

Recurrent Respiratory Papillomatosis

Recurrent respiratory papillomatosis (RRP) is a relatively rare disease caused by HPV types 6, 11, and, occasionally, 16. RRP is more common in men than women. The disease is characterized by the growth of benign finger-like projections called papillomas in the respiratory tract, particularly in the larynx (larynx is another name for the voice box; it forms the top part of the windpipe, located toward the front of the neck), and causes partial blockages of the breathing passages.

There are nearly 6,000 new cases of RRP per year in the United States. The disease peaks in two stages of life and affects both children and adults. The first peak occurs in children between two and four years of age, with approximately 2,300 new pediatric cases per year. Infants with RRP usually have a weak cry. Twenty-five percent of the cases occur during the first year of life, with boys and girls equally affected. Nearly 75 percent of affected children are firstborn vaginally delivered infants of teenage mothers. The open mouth of a newborn presents an ideal mucous membrane for HPV infection, and, when the virus enters the mouth and throat, it can produce benign wart-like growths on the larynx. Infants born through an infected birth canal seem to be more at risk than those born by Cesarean section. Not all infants delivered to mothers with

HPV infections get RRP—host factors such as a weakened immune system play an essential role in the risk of development of RRP. Active or latent HPV cervical infection is found in approximately 10–25 percent of women of childbearing age in the United States, but only 1 in 400 infants delivered to these women is estimated to be at risk for subsequent RRP.

The second peak of RRP occurs between the ages of 20 and 30 years and is believed to be sexually transmitted through oral sex, affecting more men than women by a margin of approximately three to two. Nearly 3,300 new cases in adult men are diagnosed per year in the United States. The majority of patients with respiratory papillomas present with hoarseness, while some patients may present with chronic cough or recurrent respiratory infections. Many times, these presenting symptoms lead to the misdiagnosis of asthma or bronchitis. At times, massive papillomas can block the airways and cause distressed breathing. Although RRP is a benign condition, it can sometimes undergo cancerous changes, particularly in those with compromised immune systems such as in patients who are smokers.

Surgical removal of the papillomas remains the mainstay of treatment, but as the name suggests, recurrences are common. Antiviral drugs such as Interferon have been used to slow the course of the disease, but none of the treatments is universally curative. In addition, the role of the HPV vaccine in preventing RRP has not been evaluated at this time.

In summary, RRP is a rare but potentially fatal condition. The impact of RRP on patients, their families, and the health-care system is immense. Unfortunately, despite extensive investigational studies, no cure is available for the disease. Further information about increasing awareness, prevention, cure and treatment of RRP can be obtained from the Recurrent Respiratory Papillomatosis Foundation (http://www.rrpf.org).

Mouth and Throat Cancers

In May 2007, the *New England Journal of Medicine* made headline news when it linked throat cancers to oral sex. Most people associate mouth and throat cancers with tobacco use, and rightfully so—cigarette smoking and heavy alcohol drinking are still the most important risk factors for overall head and neck cancers.

There was, however, one intriguing phenomenon that doctors observed. Despite the correlation between the dramatic decline in the rates of cigarette smoking after the 1960s (when the U.S. Surgeon General released a report that highlighted its negative effects and legislation was passed to start labeling cigarette packs) and the reduction in the overall rates of head and neck cancers, the rates of throat cancers—particularly those of the tonsils, base of the tongue and the back of the throat (also called oropharyngeal region)—did not decline, and actually appeared to be gradually rising. Cancer of the tonsils has been rising at a rate of approximately 4 percent per year and cancer of the base of the tongue has been rising at a rate of approximately 2 percent per year for the last 30 years, particularly in adults in their forties. Furthermore, 50 percent of these cancers appeared in nonsmokers. The missing link was eventually found in HPV infections, specifically infections caused by the HPV 16 strain, which partially negated the overall reduction in head and neck cancers that was gained from the decline in tobacco use.

Another clue to this enigmatic puzzle was found in a key study from the Swedish Cancer Registry in which interesting data showed that the prevalence of HPV 16 in throat cancers increased from 23 percent in the 1970s, to 28 percent in the 1980s, to 57 percent in the 1990s, and to 68 percent so far in the twenty-first century. This increase in infections has occurred simultaneously as the smoking prevalence has declined dramatically in Sweden, suggesting that an epidemic of oropharyngeal cancers associated with HPV 16 was possibly due to the current sexual practices of adolescents and adults who are engaging in more frequent oral-genital sex than ever before. Similar reasons most likely also hold true for the rising statistics in the United States.

From the above research and statistics, it can be surmised that oral sex—although less risky than genital sexual intercourse—comes with its own gamut of risks, from warts in the mouth to cancer in the throat. Like the cell lining in the cervix, the squamous epithelial lining in the mouth acts as a magnet for HPV infections. Oral sex, including fellatio (performed on a man), cunnilingus (performed on a woman), and analingus (oral to anal stimulation performed on a man or a woman) are the main transits for oral HPV infections; even though mouth to mouth transmissions can also occur.

Statistically, very few oral HPV infections lead to oropharyngeal cancers but, given the opportunity, oral HPV infections can play a significant role in the development of oropharyngeal cancers. According to the American Cancer Society, HPV may be responsible for about 20 to 30 percent of the estimated 34,360 cases of mouth and throat cancer that occurred in the United States in 2007. HPV-related throat cancer strikes about 11,000 new men and women each year. Men are three times more prone to oropharyngeal cancers than women. In addition, men have been found to have a more virulent form of mouth and throat cancer than women.

> ☞ Tobacco smoking and heavy alcohol drinking are the most significant risk factors for overall head and neck cancers. In recent times, HPV infections of the mouth have played an important role in the rise in rates of oropharyngeal cancers.

There is no test currently approved for detecting HPV in the mouth. The best way to prevent the overall incidence of oropharyngeal cancers would be to further reduce the local societal practices of tobacco smoking, chewing tobacco, and heavy drinking. In addition, safer sex practices such as delaying sexual activity, staying in a monogamous relationship, and consistently using condoms and dental dams during oral sex should be practiced. (A dental dam is a wide piece of rubbery material, usually made of latex, that one places over the vulva or anus during oral-vaginal or oral-anal sex. Dental dams help reduce transmission of bacteria and viruses from vaginal and anal fluids to the mouth. Dental dams can also be made by cutting open an unlubricated male condom.) If you do not know how to use a dental dam, do not be embarrassed. Talk to your health-care provider.

It will also be interesting to conduct studies in the future to determine if the HPV vaccine that is currently being administered to women will reduce the incidence of HPV-related oropharyngeal cancers in women. If that is the case, then there would be one more compelling reason to test the vaccine in men in order to possibly help prevent the spread of the more virulent form of oral cancer in men.

Genital Warts

The topic of genital warts has been discussed in greater detail in Chapter 4. Suffice it to say that an estimated 1 percent of all sexually active men are diagnosed with genital warts at some point in their lifetime. About 500,000 new cases of genital warts are diagnosed in men every year in the United States. Men can develop warts on any part of their genitals such as the penis, the scrotum, in and around the anus, the opening and inside of the urethra, and in and around the groin area. HIV-positive men, in particular, often have widespread recurrent warts.

Penile warts can be hard to find. Most often, they appear in areas that are subjected to friction during intercourse. In uncircumcised men, this site is usually on the inside of the foreskin, whereas, in circumcised men, it is usually on the shaft of the penis. Some experienced doctors paint the penis with vinegar (5 percent acetic acid) and look for warts under a magnifying glass. Penile warts, like other warts, are treated with topical medications. Recurrent warts sometimes have to be biopsied to rule out any underlying cancer. Unfortunately, there is no evidence to show that treating patients' penile warts actually reduces the risk of HPV transmission to their partners. Therefore "cured" patients are still at risk of transmitting the virus to their sexual partners and should use condoms.

Penile Cancers

Penile cancers are rare in men in the United States. They occur in one out of every 100,000 men in this country (CDC 2007). By and large, the single most important determining factor in the incidence of penile cancer is the proportion of the population that is circumcised. In the United States, about 60–80 percent of men are circumcised. In 2006, around

1,530 cases of penile cancer were diagnosed in men in the United States, and around 300 deaths from it. Penile cancer accounted for 0.2 percent of all cancers in men and 0.1 percent of all cancer deaths in men that year. The racial and geographic distribution of penile cancer in the United States parallels that of cervical cancer. Such an occurrence is called "geographical clustering." Penile cancer is highest among African American and Hispanic men from the South and in white men from the Appalachian regions of Kentucky and West Virginia. Higher rates of smoking, coupled with lower rates of circumcision and poor penile hygiene, are thought to be some of the causative factors.

On the other hand, penile cancer on the global front is not an insignificant problem—it affects nearly 100,000 men a year worldwide. It accounts for almost 10–20 percent of all cancers in men in countries where males are not routinely circumcised at birth. Penile cancers typically affect older men between 50 and 70 years of age. Ninety-three percent of penile cancers are squamous cell carcinomas, and 50–70 percent of penile cancer is linked to HPV infections.

Some studies have shown that circumcision at birth is associated with a threefold decrease in the risk of penile cancer; this protective effect is diminished, however, when the procedure is performed later in life. For example, in the Jewish culture, the tradition is to circumcise the male infant by the eighth day after he is born. In the Muslim culture, the procedure can wait until the tenth year of life. Similarly, in other cultures that practice circumcision—such as the Ibos of Nigeria—the incidence of penile cancer is low, as compared to those that do not, such as Hindus.

Other risk factors for penile cancer include phimosis (a condition where the foreskin becomes difficult to retract, and thus, cleaning becomes tedious), ultraviolet light treatments for the penis for a chronic skin condition called psoriasis, and herpes simplex type 2 infections of the foreskin (balanitis). In addition, some of the risk factors that lead women to develop cervical cancer, such as having multiple sex partners and unprotected sex, also increase the progression in men to penile cancer. Studies have shown that the prevalence of cervical cancer is increased three to eightfold in women whose sexual partners had penile cancer, thus elucidating the so-called "ping-pong effect" of the virus. Let us hope that the HPV vaccine for men will not only help reduce the risk of penile cancers in men but will also help reduce the risk of cervical cancer in women.

Anal Cancer in Gay, Bisexual, and HIV-Positive Men

Men having sex with men are at a high risk and HIV-positive men are at the highest risk of having persistent HPV throughout their life span. In the general population, however, *larger* numbers of women than men get anal cancer because there is a higher number of women (heterosexual and bisexual) having receptive anal sex than gay and bisexual men, who constitute a very small percentage of the population (CDC 2005). Nonetheless, gay, bisexual, and HIV-positive men are at a *higher risk* of getting anal cancer than any other segment of the society (Schottenfeld et al. 1996).

It is unfortunate that many MSM do not realize that they are at an elevated risk for anal cancer. It is estimated that the incidence of anal cancer in MSM who are HIV negative and have a history of receptive anal intercourse is approximately 35 per 100,000, the same incidence as that of cervical cancer prior to the implementation of Pap smears that promoted early detection and treatment among at-risk women. With the added burden of HIV, the incidence of anal cancer in HIV-positive men is double— 70 per 100,000, or approximately 70 times the current rate of anal cancer that is seen in the general population (1–1.5 per 100,000; refer to Table 7.2). Risk factors for anal cancer, in addition to sexual orientation and being HIV positive, include multiple partners, lack of condom use, circumcision status, history of other sexually transmitted infections, smoking more than 10 cigarettes per day, race and ethnicity, and education level. Unfortunately, there have been fewer advances in prevention of and education about HPV for gay and bisexual men. Anal cancer rates have doubled in the last 10 years and are expected to continue to rise. MSM and HIV-positive men and women have seen the sharpest increase in anal cancers, and they also have the lowest survival rates.

A study comprising 357 MSM at the University of California, San Francisco (UCSF) found that HPV-related diseases in HIV-positive men has increased in the past decade. This was particularly true of anal dysplasia, also known as anal intraepithelial neoplasia (AIN), which may be a precursor to cancer. As better drugs have caused HIV to be seen as a chronic disease as opposed to a death sentence, they may also, ironically, lead to higher rates of HPV-associated diseases in the future. Because men with HIV now live longer than before, HPV has a better chance of causing advanced diseases such as anal cancer in their lifetime (Palefsky et al. 2005). Some scientists were optimistic that, with the newer drugs for HIV, there might actually be a regression of HPV-associated lesions, but so far, all data point to that not being the case.

Cervical Pap smears dropped the rate of cervical cancer by nearly 75 percent—from 30–40 per 100,000 to 8 per 100,000. The good news is that anal cancer, like cervical cancer, is preventable and highly curable in the early stages of the disease. An anal Pap test is a test similar to a cervical Pap test, in which a sample of cells is collected from the transitional zone of the anal canal (the area where the anus and rectum meet), and examined under the microscope for any abnormal changes. The anal Pap test is inexpensive and relatively painless. One mathematical model that is based on current clinical evidence showed that if anal Pap smear screening were to be done every two to three years in HIV-negative men

Table 7.2 HPV Prevalence in the Anal Canal and Incidence of Anal Cancer in Men

Category	Approximate prevalence rate
Prevalence in HIV-negative gay men	60%–75%
Prevalence in HIV-positive men	80%–100%
Prevalence in men with multiple types of HPV, including high-risk types in HIV-negative gay men	23%
Prevalence in men with multiple types of HPV, including high-risk types in HIV-positive gay men	61%
Incidence of anal cancer in HIV-negative gay men	35/100,000 men
Incidence of anal cancer in HIV-positive gay men	70/100,000 men
Incidence of anal cancer in the general population	1–1.5/100,000 men

at high risk, such as men who receive receptive anal sex, the cost to insurance companies would be about $16,000 per year of life gained, as compared to annual mammography, which costs approximately $120,000 per year of life gained. Researchers also believe that annual or biannual anal Pap screens in the HIV-positive group would also be as cost-effective as other accepted screening measures in medicine such as cervical cancer screening using Pap tests. But, at the present time, anal Pap test, a potential screening measure, is not a part of routine care for those at risk.

> ☞ More women get anal cancers than men, but gay, bisexual, and HIV-infected men are at greater risk of getting anal cancers than the general population.

Current studies are showing that the HPV vaccine *Gardasil* significantly reduces the incidence of HPV-related anogenital diseases in young women. The hope is that if the HPV vaccine is approved in men, it may also greatly benefit in preventing HPV-related anal diseases in them as well.

CAN MEN BE TESTED FOR HPV?—HPV TESTING IN MEN

Unlike HPV testing in women, testing options in men are limited. There is currently no FDA-approved test to detect HPV in men. In addition, as many studies on HPV in men are still in their infancy, doctors are not even sure which anatomical sites to test and how. So far, urine, semen, and urethral samples have yielded very poor results for HPV. As opposed to the moist surface of the cervix in women, the dry skin of the penis offers inadequate samples. Therefore, in order to look at the optimal anatomical sites and methods for sampling for HPV in males, a study was conducted among 463 men from the years 2003 to 2006 (Giuliano et al. 2007). As bizarre as it sounds, a fine-grade sandpaper was used to loosen the cells, and the site was then rubbed with a saline moistened Dacron swab and the specimen sent to the lab for HPV DNA testing. From these samples, it was found that there was a high prevalence of HPV on the penile shaft, the glans penis (the sensitive tip of the penis, also called the "head" of the penis), and the coronal sulcus (the groove between the shaft and the glans of the penis). This was followed by its presence on the scrotum. In gay and bisexual men, anal and perianal (area surrounding the anus) samplings also showed a high prevalence of HPV (33 percent). Therefore, it is suggested that at a minimum, the penile shaft and the glans penis/ coronal sulcus should be sampled in heterosexual men. Homosexual men should also have samples obtained from the scrotum, the perianal, and the anal areas for optimal HPV detection.

HPV Vaccination for Men

HPV vaccines in men have been a part of the debate on HPV vaccination from the very start. So, should men get the vaccine? There are no definite answers—yet. But, research in men is in progress, and more concrete results should be available in the very near future.

HPV Vaccine Research in Men

HPV research in men is still in its infancy. However, there are a few clinical trials that are underway to study the natural history of HPV in men and the role the vaccines could play. It is hoped that all these data will have many practical implications in determining whether a vaccine for men is a viable option in the future, not only to prevent HPV-related diseases in men but also to determine whether they should be employed in the arsenal against cervical cancer in women. Some of the noteworthy trials are discussed here.

H. Lee Moffitt Cancer Center & Research Institute

The National Institutes of Health (NIH) has granted the H. Lee Moffitt Cancer Center & Research Institute in Tampa, Florida, $10 million to study the role of men in spreading the human papillomavirus. Two studies are concurrently in progress at the Moffitt Center. One is called the HIM study (Natural History of HPV Infections in Men study), and the other is studying the effect of the HPV vaccine in men.

Around 3,000 men from Brazil, Mexico, and the United States are enrolled in the study. The vaccine study will provide data to show if the vaccine will reduce the number of HPV infections in men and subsequently reduce the cervical cancer incidence in women.

Merck Research Laboratories

Merck is also conducting a study similar to that of the Moffitt Cancer Institute. The Merck study includes both sexually active heterosexual and homosexual men between the ages of 16 and 23. In heterosexual men, the main benefits of an HPV vaccine will be studied in the areas of prevention of genital warts and the potential to prevent cervical cancer in women, whereas in homosexual men, its main area of interest will be looking at the development of anal pathology.

Two previous Merck studies in 9- to 15-year-old boys established the vaccine's safety and found that it produced a high level of immunity in boys, similar to that found in girls. The safety and tolerance profiles for the vaccine in men were also found to be similar to those in women. However, it is not yet known whether all of these parameters actually translate to effective protection from vaccine-targeted strains of HPV infections in men.

HPV Vaccine Facts in Males

- HPV 6 and 11 cause more than 90 percent of all genital warts in men.
- HPV 16 and 18 cause 70–90 percent of anal cancers, 50–70 percent of penile cancers, and 23–36 percent of mouth and throat cancers in men.
- The U.S. Food and Drug Administration has not approved use of the HPV vaccine for boys and men in the United States. At this time there no efficacy data to demonstrate that the vaccine can protect males from getting warts or developing HPV-related cancers or protecting their female partners from cervical cancer.
- Off-label use of the vaccine is not recommended. However, some doctors, at their own discretion, are already vaccinating their high-risk patients, such as MSM and HIV-positive patients.
- Doctors in countries such as Australia, New Zealand, and Austria are vaccinating boys based on complex mathematical calculations that indicate it will reduce the incidence of cervical cancer in women.

Potential Vaccine Advantages in Men

Even though there is no conclusive evidence yet that the vaccine will be effective in men, mathematical modeling studies show that:

- If the vaccine were administered to men, it would establish overall immunity and reduce the HPV pool in circulation.
- Ninety percent of the conditions caused by HPV types 6, 11, 16, and 18 could be eliminated if girls *and* boys were vaccinated before the age of 12. Vaccinating only girls would result in only a 75 percent reduction.

- In communities or countries where there is hesitation to vaccinate girls, vaccinating boys as well will reduce the focus on women as being the sole bearers of the most common sexually transmitted disease.
- *Gardasil* may also be nearly 100 percent effective against genital warts in men. As men worry a great deal about the cosmetic appearance of warts and their disfigurement, having protection against warts may lend a cachet to getting vaccinated.
- The vaccine could be of benefit in preventing anal cancers in men because the lining of the anal canal is very similar in structure to the lining of the cervix. Phase 3 clinical trials have shown that *Gardasil* causes a 100 percent reduction in the incidence of HPV-associated anogenital diseases in young women against types 6, 11, 16, and 18.
- The HPV vaccines could be particularly useful in MSM and HIV-positive men, in whom the rates of anal cancer are 17 times and 37 times higher than that of the general population, respectively. The vaccine could be of benefit in HIV-positive men who are more prone to getting severe and prolonged cases of warts that are more resistant to treatment. Preventive vaccines work mainly through humoral immunity (refer to Chapter 6 on *Vaccines*), which is relatively well preserved in individuals with HIV in earlier stages of the disease.
- The vaccines could be of benefit in preventing penile cancers. The lining of the squamous epithelium of the penis is similar to that of the vulva, and the vaccine has already been approved for use in preventing HPV-related vulvar dysplasias.
- The vaccine could prove beneficial in preventing HPV 16– and 18–related oral cancers.

Lingering Questions about the Vaccine in Men

At this time, there are more questions than answers about HPV vaccination in men. Many compelling questions remain unanswered, some of which include the following:

- Will the HPV vaccine be as effective in men as it has proved to be in women?
  Effectiveness in women does not automatically translate to its being effective in men. Protection from the vaccine in males and females may be different because the thickness of the squamous epithelium in the genital organs varies between the two sexes. Therefore, more clinical trials are required in order to quantify the efficacy of the vaccine in men.
- If the vaccine is so effective in women, will vaccinating men only give a marginal benefit?
  It seems clear from a public policy standpoint that if a sexually transmitted disease has to be kept under check, both sexes should be involved equally in the preventive process. However, not enough data is available at this time to work out the cost-benefit ratio. This argument also does not take into consideration the risk of HPV infections among men who only have sex with men.

- Will religious beliefs hamper vaccination in boys as it has done in girls? Conservative groups believe that the vaccine in girls will promote sexual promiscuity. Similarly, when the vaccine is introduced in men, there could be fears that it may promote sexual promiscuity and homosexuality among men. Only education and knowledge will allay such fears.
- Will the vaccine give high-risk men a false sense of security and prevent them from pursuing other preventive measures, such as consistent use of condoms?
Unfortunately, this may happen, but common sense should prevail. This vaccine does not offer protection against any other STIs. The vaccine will only be an extra preventive tool, but it should not, in any way, take the place of practicing safer sex and maintaining a healthy lifestyle.
- Will HIV-positive men get full benefit from the vaccine?
Many HIV-positive men have already been infected with the types covered by the vaccine. In addition, they are often affected by multiple cancer-causing strains. Therefore, the current vaccines may not prove to be as effective in this population

> ☞ Currently, the HPV vaccine is not approved for men in the United States.

as they are in the general population. Table 7.3 gives a brief overview of HPV facts in males versus females.

EDUCATION IN MEN: A NEGLECTED FIELD

HPV has long been seen as solely a female health issue. But, as we now know, HPV is not an exclusively woman's health issue; HPV infections in men are of great importance as well. Even though for the individual man the level of risk associated with HPV infection appears to be low, targeting men will help mold future public health strategies to contain the incidence and spread of HPV infections, given that sexual transmission is the primary mode of spread to women. Including men will also take the sole focus away from women, which in conservative communities such as in India would be very welcome. Men should be equal players in the health education efforts, and emphasis should be placed on cost-effective strategies, such as consistent use of condoms, maintaining penile hygiene, and eliminating cigarette smoking. MSM and HIV-positive men should receive special attention in these efforts, as they are the segment of the population with the highest risk of infection rates. Screening, the present role of the vaccine, and future expectations should be discussed among this population. Fifty years ago, the cervical Pap smear received strong support from researchers, clinicians, and public health leaders, and that led to a dramatic decrease in the incidence of cervical cancer. A similar effort should be actively underway to target gay and bisexual men—the group most at risk for anal cancer—with anal Pap smears, particularly those who are living with HIV. But unfortunately,

Table 7.3 HPV Facts—Male versus Female: Overview

Facts	Male HPV	Female HPV
HPV infections	Less well known in men.	Have been studied since 1920.
HPV-linked diseases	Genital warts, RRP, anal, and penile cancers, and some cases of head and neck cancers.	Predominantly cervical cancer. Also genital warts, RRP vulvar, vaginal, and anal cancers.
Role in transmission	Viewed as a perpetrator for female HPV infections.	Viewed as the prey for HPV.
Screening program	None approved.	Pap smear screening since 1943. HPV DNA testing in women over 30.
HPV Testing	None approved.	HPV testing—Hybrid capture and PCR approved.
Health education	Men not included.	Only targets women.
Treatment	Only symptomatic.	Treatment of symptoms including follow-up of Pap smears.
Cure	None.	None.
Prevention	Condoms, about 70% effective. Circumcision and good penile hygiene helpful. Healthy lifestyle.	Vaccine now approved to cover types 6, 11, 16, and 18. Healthy lifestyle.

there is a disturbing lack of large-scale studies and research funding for anal cancer prevention, and issues such as stigma, politics, and low profit margins for drug companies have hampered progress. And, even though the answers are thornier than the questions, the truth remains that focusing on women alone is not going to address the issue of HPV-related diseases. The elusive "male factor" has to be addressed in order to eradicate the viral load from society and protect the health of women. If not, genital HPV infections will continue to be a serious problem.

Let me conclude with what Darron Brown, MD, professor of medicine, microbiology, and immunology at the Indiana University School of Medicine in Indianapolis, had to say: "When you want to reduce disease in a population, you immunize as many people as you can. If you can immunize a large percentage of men and prevent them from infecting women, you can reduce the disease in women."

Key Facts

- HPV 6 and 11 cause 90 percent of genital warts.
- HPV 16 and 18 cause 80–90 percent of anal cancers and 50 percent of penile cancers in men.
- HPV vaccines are not currently approved for boys and men in the United States.
- Consistent use of condoms can reduce HPV transmission by 70 percent.
- Circumcised men have a lower rate of HPV infections.
- Tobacco smoking is one of the major risk factors for HPV infections and HPV-related cancers in males.
- Focusing on women alone does not fully address the issue of HPV-related disease. Men should be equal players in reducing the viral load in society.
- When the vaccines become available to men, they will only serve as an additional layer to the preventive strategies adopted to lessen HPV infections. They *will not and should not* take the place of practicing safer sex and maintaining a healthy lifestyle.

8

FAQ's on HPV and the Vaccines: Excerpts From a University Town Hall Meeting

The introduction of the HPV vaccine on college campuses has been accompanied by healthy doses of both good and bad news. The good news is that the vaccine's arrival has brought the virus into the spotlight by giving it the press it deserves. In this instance, the pharmaceutical company's aggressive campaign efforts to market its product in the commercial realm may actually have brought a positive impact on public health education—if not for clarity, at least for the issue. But the bad news is that myths and misconceptions abound, and these can cause considerable harm. One can go through undue anxiety, have unnecessary treatment that could have been avoided, and, most dangerous of all, neglect a simple procedure that could have saved a life.

This lack of public awareness is certainly a discredit to my medical profession. With the enthusiastic marketing of the vaccine, many women on college campuses now think that cervical cancer is a common disease that can be fully prevented by the vaccine. This lack of broad understanding about the HPV family and the HPV vaccine is extremely important to address, because safer sex and healthy lifestyle choices are still crucial precautions to take against HPV even if one chooses to get the vaccine.

In an effort to put an end to the campus folklore and the irrational health concern among the college populace, I took an opportunity to address interested students at a university campus about the subject. Most students who attended these meetings had some prior knowledge of HPV. Due to this, some of the very basics of HPV were not covered in this forum, but a discussion covering the fundamentals is provided in Chapter 1. The audience comprised mainly women, but a few interested men were also present.

What follows is a compilation of questions that I encountered on the topic of genital HPV and the vaccine from the 17–24-year-old age group. In addition, I have also included questions that have often been posed by my patients individually to me in my clinical practice setting over the years. The majority of the questions that came from the college-aged group focused mainly on HPV infections and birth control pills, HPV and its effect on future pregnancies, and the efficacy of the vaccine in the college-aged population. Cost was also a big concern, as was living with a sexually transmitted infection that is silent, incurable, transmitted freely, and can resurface without warning. This dialogue with the college-aged population made the discussions interesting and helped turn what could have been a dry collection of statistics into a vibrant arc of interactive discussion. By weeding out the persistent offenders of bad information, it made room for more accurate information to take root and grow.

Q: How common is HPV?
A: HPV, or the human papillomavirus, is the most common sexually transmitted infection. It is estimated that about 20 million people in the United States are currently infected with it. Over 6 million new cases of HPV infections are diagnosed each year. Eight out of every 10 men and women who have ever had sex will get HPV at some time in their lives. HPV is most common in young men and women who are in their late teens or early twenties. The majority of HPV infections cause no symptoms. Most infections clear up on their own in 12–24 months without causing any symptoms.

Q: How does one get HPV infections? Is HPV spread only by sex?
A: Sexual intercourse is the most common way to transmit genital HPV. However, this is not the only way. HPV can be spread by sexual contact without intercourse, such as foreplay and skin contact with the labia, penis, and inner thigh. In addition, warts on the hands and feet (which are caused by low-risk HPV and do not cause genital warts) are spread by coming in contact with infected surfaces. HPV can also be spread from mother to child during childbirth. Infected mothers can pass the virus to their babies when they are passing through the birth canal and cause warts in the baby's eyes and airways. Fortunately, these conditions are extremely rare.

The biggest risk for getting HPV, however, comes from engaging in high-risk sexual behavior such as having multiple partners (Manhart et al. 2006), having unprotected sex, and starting to have sex at an early age. In addition, having a weak immune system due to poor nutrition, stress, or taking certain types of medications such as steroids can all nurture HPV infections.

Q: Can two people in a monogamous relationship get HPV?
A: The short answer to the above question is, unfortunately, yes. Because the majority of sexual partners presently in a monogamous relationship

may have had prior sexual partners, and because HPV can lie dormant in the human body for many years before becoming active, contracting HPV is certainly a possibility. The only way to prevent HPV from sexual contact is for both partners in a monogamous relationship to have never had prior sexual partners.

Q: HPV and cervical cancer—what is the connection?
A: Ninety-nine percent of cervical cancers are caused by HPV (Walboomers et al. 1999). However, there are *very few* HPV infections that lead to cervical cancer. For example, there are about 20 million people with HPV infections at any given time in the United States. About 6.2 million cases of HPV infection occur every year (Weinstock et al. 2004). Approximately 11,000 women end up getting cervical cancer every year, and about 4,000 of those die from it. Even though the 4,000 deaths are 4,000 too many, the ratio of cervical cancer to HPV infections in the United States is very small. This is due to the implementation of successful widespread screening programs such as the Pap test that help with early detection and treatment.

Q: I have heard that there many types of HPV. Do they all cause cervical cancer?
A: There are over 100 types of HPV. Out of those, there are a little over a dozen that have the potential to cause cervical cancer. These are called high-risk types. The other types of HPVs that do not cause cancer are called low/intermediate types. Examples of these types are those that cause genital warts. However, even high-risk HPV infections rarely lead to cancer. The immune systems of most women will usually suppress or spontaneously clear the virus.

Q: How long does it take for one to progress from HPV infections to cervical cancer?
A: First of all, very few HPV infections progress to cervical cancer, as most infections resolve on their own. Only a handful of infections progress through the different stages of HPV acquisition, HPV persistence, development of precancerous lesions, and invasive cancer. The whole process usually takes 20 years on average, with the longest duration being between the precancerous stage and invasive cancer. A few cases, however, develop more rapidly, but this is rare.

Q: What is the prognosis for cervical cancer?
A: The prognosis for cervical cancer depends on the stage at which it is diagnosed. The earlier the stage, the better the five-year survival rate. (A five-year survival rate refers to the percentage of patients who live at least five years after their cancer diagnosis is made. This percentage serves as a standard way to discuss a patient's prognosis in general.) The five-year survival rate for cervical cancer ranges from 96–99 percent for the early stages of the disease, to 15–20 percent for the late stages of the disease (ACS).

Q: Can HPV skip precancerous stages and develop straight into cervical cancer?
A: Yes, but those instances are very rare. HPV infections can progress to cancer much faster in those who are HIV positive and/or have a very weak immune system.

Q: Does the HPV vaccine prevent cervical cancer?
A: The vaccine currently available in the United States, *Gardasil* made by Merck, protects against four HPV types—6, 11, 16, and 18. Types 16 and 18 are the cancer-causing types that, together, are responsible for 70 percent of cervical cancers. Types 6 and 11 cause genital warts. The second vaccine currently awaiting approval in the United States is *Cervarix* made by GlaxoSmithKline. It, too, covers HPV types 16 and 18. Therefore, both the vaccines give protection against 70 percent of cervical cancers. In order to maximize protection against all HPVs, regular Pap tests are strongly recommended to detect the remaining 30 percent of cervical cancers. It is well worth repeating this extremely salient point: *the vaccines provide protection against only 70 percent of cervical cancers, so regular Pap smears are still required to detect the remaining 30 percent of cervical cancers.*

Q: What are the causes for the other 30 percent of cervical cancers?
A: The majority of the other 30 percent is caused by HPV types not covered by the vaccine. A very small percentage, less than 1 percent, occurs due to other causes not yet well understood.

Q: Can HPV cause other types of cancer?
A: Yes. Apart from cervical cancer, HPV can cause vaginal, vulvar, anal, penile, and some head and neck cancers.

Q: Does the vaccine protect against other cancers?
A: So far, the vaccine has also been approved for protection against vulvar and vaginal precancerous lesions caused by HPV types 16 and 18.

Q: Does the vaccine protect against other sexually transmitted infections?
A: NO, the vaccine does not protect against other STIs. Therefore, limiting one's number of sexual partners and using barrier methods such as male or female condoms and dental dams on a consistent basis is still encouraged.

Q: When is the ideal time to get the vaccine and why?
A: As the vaccine is preventive, the ideal time to get the vaccine is before sexual debut, or before it is possible for any HPV infections to be contracted. The CDC recommends that the best time to get the vaccine is between the ages of 11 and 12 years. Statistics show that approximately 13 percent of students are sexually active by the time they are 15 years old, and nearly 50 percent are sexually active by the time they graduate from high school (CDC 2002). Therefore, 11–12 years old seems to be an ideal time to vaccinate before most children become sexually active. In addition, drop-out rates from school start increasing as children

approach high school. So 11–12 years old may be the last chance to administer the vaccine along with other vaccines such as the DTaP (Diphtheria Tetanus and acellular Pertussis) vaccine and Meningococcal vaccine. The vaccine can also be administered to females as young as nine years and as old as 26 years.

Q: Is it true that the vaccine is not as effective when given to college-aged women?

A: As mentioned before, the vaccine is preventive. Surveys show that 70 percent of college women are already sexually active. Therefore, they may have already been exposed to the HPV types covered by the vaccine. Recent studies show that both vaccines are 98–100 percent effective against HPV types 16 and 18 when a woman is not exposed to the vaccine-covered HPV types. However, once she becomes sexually active, the efficacy of the vaccine drops to 44 percent (*FUTURE II* studies).

Q: If the vaccine is recommended before sexual debut and not as effective in college-aged females, why is this age group still being targeted aggressively?

A: Even though 70 percent of women in college are already sexually active, the remaining 30 percent are not. Therefore, the women who are not yet sexually active will fully benefit today from the vaccine. In addition, others who are already sexually active may have just started having sex, or may not yet have been exposed to all the types that the vaccine covers. This is the reason why "catch-up" vaccinations are recommended for females aged 13–26, based on their sexual history and their potential benefit from vaccination.

Q: Some people believe that the vaccine would promote sexual promiscuity if given to 11–12-year olds. What are your thoughts on this?

A: No, the vaccine will not promote sexual promiscuity. In fact, it will serve as a platform to educate teenagers about HPV infections and other STIs. Sexual behavior in young men and women is influenced by many factors such as the fear of pregnancy and acquiring HIV. Contracting HPV or any other STI does not seem to be on the top of the list. It should also be pointed out that the HPV vaccine does not prevent against other STIs, such as HIV, gonorrhea, and chlamydia. Therefore, it seems unlikely that getting the vaccine would lead teenagers to believe that they could have sex without any possible negative consequences.

Q: Will the vaccine give a false sense of security to those who get it?

A: It might, but that should not be the case. *Gardasil*, the vaccine that is currently available in the United States, only protects against two strains of HPV that cause cancer and two strains of HPV that cause genital warts. As previously mentioned, there are more than a dozen oncogenic forms of HPV. Hence, a regular Pap test schedule as recommended by your healthcare provider should be followed. In addition, educating the public about HPV infections and the role of vaccines will be of paramount importance.

Q: How long will the vaccine stay effective after I get it?
A: So far, clinical trials have shown both of the vaccines to be effective for at least 5 years (Villa et al. 2006). As trials continue over time, we may find that the vaccines are effective for a longer period of time.

Q: If the vaccine trials have been in progress for only five years, and it takes an average of 20 years for cervical cancer to develop, how can we conclude that the vaccine will prevent cervical cancer?
A: Great question. To be honest, the medical community is currently taking a leap of faith to some extent. No one will really know for another 25–40 years if the vaccine truly prevents cervical cancer, because all the 11–12-year-old girls who are being vaccinated today have to approach the ages of 35–50, the age range when cervical cancer peaks.

However, having said that, there is enough scientific evidence to support the theory that the vaccines can prevent cervical cancer. Clinical trials look at cancer surrogates, or conditions which when left alone will invariably progress to invasive cervical cancer, as end points of the study. For example, they currently look for significantly abnormal cells on Pap smears called CIN II/CIN III cervical dysplasias in women who have been vaccinated. These conditions develop within a few years after HPV infections. The vaccines have been found to prevent the development of these abnormal lesions. So, it has been hypothesized that the vaccines will prevent cervical cancer.

Q: If I get the vaccine, will it cause me to get a mild form of the infection or cancer? Will I test positive for HPV in the future?
A: No. This is a unique vaccine. Unlike vaccines in the past, this one does not contain a killed or a weakened version of the virus. Therefore, it cannot cause infection or cancer. Nor can you test positive for HPV.

Q: Then how does the vaccine work?
A: The vaccine is made from a protein called the L1 protein that is found on the envelope of the virus. When assembled in a particular fashion, these L1 proteins are believed to trick the immune system of the body into thinking that they are the real virus and stimulate it to produce antibodies against the vaccine types. Thus, when the real virus attacks, there is plenty of antibodies to fight it. Both the vaccines are made from the L1 proteins.

Q: What are the side effects from the vaccine?
A: The most common side effect is pain at the site of injection—8 out of 10 women who receive the vaccine complain of it. Swelling and redness at the injected site is the second most common side effect.

For more details on side effects, refer to Chapter 6.

Q: How much does the vaccine cost?
A: The vaccine costs around $120 for each shot in the three-shot series, plus administration fees.

Q: The vaccine is very expensive. Can I just get one shot?
A: So far, the efficacy of the vaccine has been studied only in those who received all three shots according to the protocol. Anything less will probably not evoke the required immune response to protect you from the targeted HPV types.

Q: Will insurance companies provide reimbursement for the vaccine?
A: Insurance coverage provided by various companies varies. As a general rule, if your insurance covers other vaccines, then it will most likely cover the HPV vaccine too. Check with your insurance company to verify coverage.

Q: Where can I get the vaccine?
A: You should be able to get the vaccine at your college health services or at your primary care doctor's office. If not, ask them where you can get the vaccine. If you do not have insurance, contact your local health department or the community health center in your area. The administrators there can help you find places that will give the vaccine to you at low cost or no cost. If you are 18 or younger and are uninsured, Medicaid eligible, Native Alaskan, or American Indian, you can get the vaccine for free through the Vaccine for Children (VFC) program. A nominal administrative fee may apply. Merck also has a patient assistance program for uninsured adults. If you are employed, you may be able to take advantage of your company health insurance's flexible spending account and get a tax deduction for the price of the vaccine.

Q: Will vaccination against the targeted HPV types cause non-vaccine HPV types to mutate and become more dangerous?
A: Viruses are extremely resilient and have great survival skills. There is a small chance that adverse mutations can occur. However, such events are rare.

Q: Will the vaccine be less effective if I have other types of HPV that are not covered by the vaccine?
A: The presence of other types of HPV will not weaken the effectiveness of the vaccine.

Q: What is the vaccine schedule?
A: The *Gardasil* vaccine is a series of three shots. The second is given two months after the first, and the third is given four months after the second. The shots are administered in the arm.

Q: I have already had my first shot last month. I am supposed to get the second one next month, but I am going to be away. What can I do?
A: The current recommendation is that you *do not* have to restart the vaccine series even if you are unable to follow the usual protocol. The CDC has recommended an alternate schedule. You can get the second shot as early as 4 weeks after the first shot. If this is not possible, get it soon after you get back.

Q: I received my second shot three months ago. I am graduating next week and will not have insurance for a while. I prefer to get the vaccine at the college health services, even though I know according to the vaccine schedule I have to wait for one more month. What can I do?

A: The third vaccine has to be spaced at least 12 weeks from the second. So, it will be acceptable for you to get the vaccine before graduating.

Q: I missed my third vaccine last semester. What is your suggestion?

A: Even though the third vaccine is supposed to be given 6 months after the first and 4 months after the second, if you miss those dates, get it as soon as possible. It is suggested that the series be completed ideally within 6 months and preferably within one year of the first shot.

Q: I am planning on being sexually active soon. I am going to receive my first HPV shot next week. How soon after the shot will I develop immunity?

A: You will get maximum benefit one month after receiving the third shot. This is when the full antibody response would have developed. But always remember to use condoms and other barrier methods as a preventive measure against HPV and other STIs.

Q: Can the HPV shot be given with other immunization vaccines?

A: Yes, the HPV vaccine can be administered with other vaccines.

Q: I got my first shot not knowing I was pregnant. What should I do?

A: First of all, do not panic. Just wait to get the rest of the shots after delivery. There is no indication that the shots cause any birth defects, so there is no reason to terminate the pregnancy. However, the vaccine pregnancy registry at the CDC should be notified if exposure to the vaccine occurs during pregnancy.

Q: Can HPV be transmitted from mother to child?

A: HPV infections can be transmitted from a mother to a child. The risk is real but rare. The baby may contract the virus during its passage through the birth canal and develop warts on the eyes and air passages. Delivery by cesarean section offers some protection, but there are no guarantees. Therefore, pregnant women should talk to their health-care professionals about individual risks and delivery options.

Q: What is the maximum age that one can receive the vaccine?

A: *Gardasil* has currently been approved for women until the age of 26 because it has been tested only up to that age. If a woman has not had sexual intercourse or has had very few sexual encounters by age 26, she can still be protected by the vaccine. Studies have shown that women of this age group put up good immune response to the vaccine. Clinical trials are now in progress to see if the vaccine would help older women. Currently, *Cervarix* has been approved outside the United States for women until the age of 45.

Q: I am hesitant to get the vaccine because it has only been out for a little over two years. What long-term side effects should I be worried about?
A: Like other vaccines or medications, it is hard to foresee every single side effect. So far, the vaccines have not shown any signs of untoward long-term side effects.

Q: I am not going to have sex until I am in a committed relationship. Do I still need the vaccine?
A: The vaccine (*Gardasil*) will prevent infections from four different HPV strains, two of which cause 90 percent of genital warts and two of which cause most cervical cancers. The vaccine will confer protection against these types in the event there is an unforeseen circumstance such as sexual assault. Such an event assumes the highest risk, and you can protect yourself to some extent if you choose to get the vaccine. You are also prone to contracting HPV if your partner has had previous sexual experience and may now be a carrier. Hence, you may still benefit from getting the vaccine.

Q: I have heard that it's harder for a woman to give HPV to a man than vice-versa. Is there any truth to this?
A: Yes, that is true. Women have a larger surface area of moist genital skin and mucus membranes than men, making them more vulnerable to HPV infections.

Q: If HPV is a sexually transmitted disease, why shouldn't men also get the vaccine?
A: It is a known fact that men also carry HPV, but most of the disease burden is carried by women. Therefore, the vaccine was first tested in women. The vaccine is currently being tested in men, and we should have the results soon.

Q: I hear HPV can be spread by oral sex. Is that true?
A: Yes, HPV can spread to the genitals and anal area during oral sex; conversely the reverse is also true. Though rare, HPV can cause warts and cancers of the mouth. About 30 percent of head and throat cancers are now attributed to HPV. It has also been found that, even though the rates of smoking and drinking have come down, the rate of throat cancers has been gradually going up. This rise has been attributed to increased rates of HPV infections from oral sex.

Q: Should men who have sex with men (MSM) get the vaccine?
A: Although the HPV vaccine has not been approved for men in the United States yet, some doctors are administering it off label (without FDA approval) to high-risk patients such as gay and bisexual men and HIV-positive patients. MSM who receive anal sex are 17 times more likely to get HPV infections when compared to heterosexual men. Being HIV positive puts gay men at even higher risks for HPV infections and anal cancers (Schottenfeld et al. 1996). Clinical trials are in progress to see if the vaccine will also be of benefit against anal cancers in both sexes.

Q: Do women who have sex with women (WSW) need the vaccine?

A: WSW are at the same risk or an even greater risk of getting HPV infections. Some may acquire it through skin-to-skin contact or contact with sex toys, while others may have bisexual relationships. In addition, many women who have sex with women only do not receive Pap tests on a regular basis, either because they believe they do not need them or because their health-care provider is poorly informed. A regularly scheduled Pap test is a smart health measure for all gay, bisexual, and straight women alike.

Q: Do condoms prevent HPV?

A: Condoms are not as effective in preventing HPV infections as they are in preventing other STIs such as gonorrhea and chlamydia. This is because HPV can also be spread by skin-to-skin contact from areas not covered by condoms such as the scrotum, inner thighs, and anal area. However, recent studied have shown that most HPV resides in areas covered by the condom such as the shaft of the penis and the head (tip) of the penis. Condoms have been found to protect up to 70 percent of HPV infections (Winer et al. 2006). Female condoms give even better protection as they cover a wider area. Despite this, they are not as frequently used as male condoms.

Q: Is it true that using birth control pills increases the risk of HPV infections?

A: There is a very small chance that birth control pills may increase the risk of HPV infections. The increased risk has been seen in young women who started taking birth control pills before the age of 20 and those who have taken them for more than 5 years (Moreno et al. 2002). However, those who started taking the pills at 20 or sooner for birth control reasons are more likely to engage in high-risk sexual behaviors such as multiple partners and unprotected sex. For those who have taken the pill for more than 5 years, it is believed that the chronic influence of the hormone estrogen, present in the birth control pills, makes the cervix more vulnerable to HPV and other STIs, but the risk is *small*. (Refer to Chapter 3 for more details.)

Q: Does smoking make one more prone to HPV infections? If so, how?

A: Smoking weakens the immune system and increases your chances of acquiring and retaining HPV infections. It has been shown that persistent HPV infections are one of the main reasons for the development of abnormal cells in the cervix (cervical dysplasia) and cervical cancer. Also, nicotine and other gases that are released while smoking are toxic to the cells and promote abnormal growth. In addition, the more cigarettes you smoke, the higher the risk. Studies have also shown that smokers who have HPV infections are at a significantly increased risk of developing cervical cancer than those who are similarly infected with HPV but do not smoke (Gunnell et al. 2006). (Refer to Chapter 3 for a more detailed explanation.)

Q: How can I find out if I have HPV?

A: There are two ways to know if you have HPV—indirect and direct. The indirect method is the Pap test. A Pap test is a very good screening test that is used to detect any abnormal changes in the cells of the cervix. The direct test is called the HPV DNA test. This test looks for the presence of HPV genetic material and not for the virus *per se*. It tests for all the high-risk HPV types as a group. Therefore, you may get a report that says "high-risk HPV present" and not specifically which HPV type. The HPV test can be performed at the same time the Pap smear is obtained. Currently, there is no HPV test approved for men.

Q: Do Pap smears pick up all HPV changes? In other words, how accurate are Pap tests?

A: Pap tests are not 100 percent accurate. In fact they are only 50–80 percent accurate. The effectiveness of a Pap smear lies in its *repetition*. Therefore, if it misses HPV changes the first time, it will pick them up the second or the third time. That is why Pap smears have to be done on a regular basis: in order to improve the accuracy. This may sound highly unscientific and based on a "hit or miss" theory, but it is important to remember that cervical cancer is a very slow-growing cancer and repeated Pap tests will pick up the abnormal cells well ahead of time in almost all cases. Therefore, Pap tests, in spite of not being very accurate, are still very good screening tests. They are inexpensive and help with early detection of a condition for which there is treatment available.

Q: How accurate is HPV DNA testing? Why isn't it more commonly used?

A: HPV DNA testing is much more accurate than Pap tests. It picks up over 90 percent of HPV infections. However, HPV DNA testing is a very expensive test and over 90 percent of HPV infections resolve on their own in people in their twenties anyway. Therefore, it would make no practical sense to perform the test in this age group where most of the infections clear up spontaneously. That is why the routine use for HPV DNA test is reserved for those over the age of 30, when the HPV infections tend to be more persistent.

Q: I am 22 years old. My Pap result earlier in the year came back abnormal. I am also positive for high-risk HPV. Does that mean I will get cancer?

A: No, that does not mean you will get cancer. All it means is that you have been exposed to one or more types of cancer-causing HPV. In an overwhelming number of cases, the abnormality is not cancerous. In addition, you have a greater than 90 percent chance of clearing the virus naturally if you practice safer sex and follow a healthy lifestyle. You will most likely be tested in 6 to 12 months to see if the virus has gone away. If your repeat Pap test remains abnormal, your health-care professional may recommend follow-up testing or procedures.

Q: Do genital warts lead to cervical cancer?

A: No, genital warts do not lead to cancer. Ninety percent of genital warts are caused by HPV 6 and 11 (Greer et al. 1995). These are not high-risk types and therefore are not cancer causing.

Q: How are genital warts treated?

A: There are several methods to treat genital warts. The most common methods are to either freeze or burn them with chemicals. This is done at your health-care professional's office. Lately, newer topical treatments have become available, and these can be applied in the privacy of your home. (Refer to Chapter 4 for more details on treatment of genital warts.)

Q: I was treated for genital warts last year. Will I still be able to transmit the HPV after treatment?

A: There is no clear answer to this. HPV transmission is still a mystery. The virus can lie dormant for years and transmit freely. There is still no convincing scientific evidence that treating genital warts reduces the rate of transmission. However, common sense dictates that when a person has an active lesion, the viral load is high in the area of the lesion and therefore extra precaution (such as condoms and other barrier methods) should be exercised to minimize transmission.

Q: I have genital warts. Should I still get the vaccine?

A: If you have had genital warts, it means you have probably been exposed to either HPV type 6 or 11 or both, because they cause 90 percent of genital warts. However, you may or may not have been exposed to types 16 and 18, which are the cancer-causing types. Therefore, the vaccine, *Gardasil*, might still protect you against types that you have not already been exposed to. The other vaccine, *Cervarix*, which is scheduled to be approved soon by the FDA, protects only against types 16 and 18 and not against genital warts.

Q: I am currently being treated for an abnormal Pap smear due to high-risk HPV. Should I still get the vaccine?

A: It is tough to tell which specific high-risk HPV type caused your abnormal Pap test. There are over a dozen high-risk types, and the HPV DNA test only looks for them as a class and not for specific ones. The vaccine protects for more than one high-risk type. *Gardasil* also protects against HPV types that cause most genital warts. Hence, you may still benefit from receiving the vaccine.

Q: I was diagnosed with HPV last week. Does that mean my partner has been cheating on me?

A: Being diagnosed with an HPV infection does *not* mean that your partner has been cheating on you. He or she might have acquired it from a previous relationship. HPV can lie dormant for years and resurface itself at any time, particularly if your immune system is weakened. (Please refer to Chapter 5 for a detailed description of the emotional aspects of HPV.)

Q: What do I tell my partner?

A: Be honest. You may want to let your partner know that HPV is a very common virus and most people do not even know they have it. HPV usually goes away by itself in one to two years. Take some educational material with you to discuss it with him or her. It might also be a good idea for your partner to talk to his or her health-care professional.

Q: If I have an abnormal Pap, should my partner get tested?
A: If your partner is a male, then there are no HPV tests approved yet. Besides, even if he has HPV, there is no way to treat him for the virus unless he has genital warts or other HPV-related visible lesions. I, however, recommend to my patients that their partners be checked by their health-care professionals. This also gives then an avenue to gain more knowledge about the infection. The CDC does not recommend examination of sexual partners at this time. On the other hand, if your partner is a female, then she should keep up her regular Pap test schedule.

Q: My boyfriend's previous partner had HPV. Should he get the vaccine?
A: Currently, the vaccine is not approved for men in the United States. However, he could reduce transmission to you by using condoms and other barrier methods at all times. Though the FDA has not approved the use of the vaccine in boys and men, some doctors are administering the vaccine on a case-by-case basis.

Q: Will a prior HPV infection confer protection against future ones?
A: In the case of HPV infections, it is still not known if natural infections provide adequate immunity to prevent future infections with the same types. The HPV vaccine has shown to evoke an antibody response that is 10-fold stronger than that evoked by a natural infection for the specific types it covers.

Q: Is there a treatment for the HPV infection?
A: Yes, HPV infections can be treated, but being treated is not the same thing as being cured. Treatments are available for warts and abnormal Pap smears. There is currently no cure for HPV infections.

Q: Is there any ongoing research to find a cure for HPV?
A: Yes, there is research going on in the development of antiviral medications against HPV infections. The role of dietary supplements such as vitamin A, folic acid, and a compound found in broccoli are all currently being investigated. In any case, having a healthy balanced meal with ample fruits and vegetables is always beneficial.

Q: Is there a way to find out if the virus has completely left the body?
A: No, there is no way to test if the virus has left the body. All that the test will tell you is that you do not currently have an active high-risk HPV infection. The test cannot detect past infections or the presence of any dormant virus residing in your body.

Q: Are there any future vaccines being developed to prevent and treat HPV infections?

A: Yes. Early clinical trials are underway to develop HPV vaccines that prevent and treat HPV infections. However, therapeutic vaccines pose an even greater challenge than the preventive vaccines. My guess is it will take at least another five to ten years before there are any therapeutic vaccines. Both Merck and GSK (the manufacturers of the HPV vaccines) are currently also trying to improve their vaccines to cover more HPV types, and these might be available sooner.

Q: If I get the current form of vaccine before the newer and better ones come out, will I need those too?

A: Currently, there are no protocols in place for future vaccines. However, it is reasonable to assume that the newer vaccines will have protection against more types of HPV infections and will also, it is hoped, treat existing HPV infections. So, you will have to consult your health-care professionals in the future to get their recommendations on the new HPV vaccines.

Q: What is the best way to prevent HPV infections?

A: The only way to prevent HPV infections is to abstain from any type of sexual activity. As this is not a practical solution for most people, being in an honest-partner commitment, postponing sexual activity, and consistently using condoms and other barrier methods can help minimize the risk of exposure to HPV. Remember the ABCDEs of minimizing HPV infections: **A**bstinence, **B**eing monogamous, consistent **C**ondom use, **D**elaying sexual activity, **E**ducation.

Q: Can cervical cancer be prevented without getting the vaccination?

A: Regular screenings can help detect nearly 100 percent of cervical cancer precursors. With timely detection and treatment, one can prevent the development of cervical cancer in most cases. The vaccines, however, will provide an added layer of protection against 70 percent of cervical cancers. Thus, the combination of the vaccine and regular cervical screening will be the best combination to prevent this devastating disease.

Key Facts

- Whereas HPV infections are very common, cervical cancer is very rare in the United States.

- HPV vaccines do not protect against other STIs. Therefore, all precautions to reduce exposure, including consistent use of condoms and other barrier methods, are recommended.

- HPV vaccines will *not* eliminate the need for regular cervical screening tests such as Pap tests because they only protect against 70 percent of cervical cancers.

- The public needs more education about the nature of HPV infections and the importance of regular cervical cancer screening.

9

PARENT'S DILEMMA TO VACCINATE: A PHYSICIAN MOTHER'S PERSPECTIVE

Myth: HPV vaccines will promote sexual promiscuity if administered to 11–12-year-old girls.

Fact: The HPV vaccines will not promote sexual promiscuity because they do not protect against pregnancy or other STIs.

We humans are undeniably products of our past. We frame our decisions and opinions based on our past experiences, biases, and cultural and religious beliefs. Oftentimes, we rely heavily on our emotions while seemingly ignoring the more salient, practical points of an argument. When it comes to decisions involving the HPV vaccine, one can certainly empathize with parents' inner conflicts as they weigh their options on whether to vaccinate their young daughters against a *sexually* transmitted disease. This is even truer when one takes into consideration that the young girls in question are only 11 and 12 years old, and they are at little or no risk of acquiring cervical cancer in the short term (cervical cancer is a very slow-growing process that typically peaks between the ages of 35 and 50 years). What an utter dilemma: On the one hand, the HPV vaccine will undoubtedly save lives; on the other hand, opposition to this new vaccine is quite pervasive and represents yet another chapter in the long history of humans' resistance to new vaccines.

The decision to vaccinate or not is seldom an easy decision for many parents. We, as a society, are generally more comfortable reacting to something rather than planning for it. We are much better at funding treatment of symptoms rather than paying for the cheaper option of preventive care. And finally, we are more comfortable taking actions that lead to short-term tangible benefits rather than implementing plans that provide life-long benefits that are not immediately identifiable.

Some parents have objections to "foreign" materials being injected into their perfectly healthy children on the off chance that the side effects from the vaccine may be worse than the disease itself. After all, a vaccine—like any other medicine—has a statistically miniscule possibility of causing an adverse reaction, and this chance may seem too risky to a parent when the immediate benefit of a vaccine is not clear to them. Another factor contributing to the hesitance of parents to subject their children to the HPV vaccine is the dramatic increase in the number of recommended vaccinations in recent years. Nowadays, children are immunized against a dozen diseases with nearly 30 shots by the time they are five years old. This stands in contrast to the three or four vaccinations children received in the 1960s and 1970s. Another contributing factor is the perceived link between these numerous vaccinations and illnesses that some people believe they may cause, such as autism, cancer, and autoimmune diseases. Some parents are convinced that many vaccines are riskier than the disease they prevent; this along with the advent of the Internet has given parents access to detailed (and often inaccurate) information that arms them with arguments even against the medical experts in the field.

In order to navigate through the numerous emotional and factual land mines that this topic presents, let us discuss the indisputable facts and see if an obvious recommendation emerges that is more palatable for everyone. Despite the numerous pros and cons of vaccines in general, it is impossible not to acknowledge the success of vaccines when you review history and realize the amazing impact that they have had in saving millions of lives around the globe. Vaccines have been one of the greatest discoveries of science in the twentieth century, and widespread aggressive immunization campaigns have largely eradicated debilitating diseases such as smallpox and polio. Yet, when it comes to the introduction of an effective vaccine targeted primarily against a sexually transmitted disease; a vaccine that must be administered to 11- and 12-year-old girls, parents face a dilemma and science faces an uphill battle.

One wonders why parents and adults would not want to protect their children and themselves from the potential ravages of cancer. Obviously, the answer to this question is complex. As a mother, I understand the various concerns that parents have, but as a physician, I have the advantage of making an educated decision based upon the knowledge and scientific data that we now have available on HPV infections and the new vaccine. It is easy for me to say, "Yes, vaccinate!" or "No, don't!" but these emphatic mandates are not nearly as powerful as giving you, the reader, the resources you need to empower and inform yourself. So, let us explore some facts and issues so that you are better prepared to answer the question for yourself later in this chapter.

Because the CDC informs us that the vaccine is most effective when administered before sexual debut, it makes sense for us to start by looking at trends in teen sexuality in the United States, so that we can honestly come to terms with the reality of the situation.

SEXUAL PRACTICES OF TEENS IN THE UNITED STATES

Human sexuality manifests itself very early in life, starting with childhood curiosity and heightening during adolescence. Adolescence is the time when dramatic hormonal and bodily changes influence teens to take risks and challenge their parents' authority and moral values. It is also the time when teens are heavily influenced by peer pressure, reproductive health education, and the all-pervasive, sexually suggestive media. Sexuality is a vital aspect of adolescent life, but it is a magnet for hysteria, conflicts, and controversies in many societies, including the United States. Such sex-negative societal attitudes lead adolescents to feel marginalized and hide their sexual lives from adults, thus making it difficult to obtain any kind of accurate information on their sexual behavior. Unfortunately, this then places them at increased health risks for unintended pregnancies and sexually transmitted infections and diseases. In spite of these obstacles, the CDC along with many other agencies and organizations such as The Kaiser Family Foundation, the National Survey of Family Growth (NSFG), and the Guttmacher Institute has collected the facts regarding teen sexual behavior in the United States. Following are approximate figures from surveys conducted by them:

- General Sexual Activity:
  - Thirteen percent of American teens are sexually experienced by the time they are 15 years old, and 70 percent are sexually experienced by 19 years of age.
  - Fourteen percent of sexually active high school students have had four or more sex partners before graduation.
  - Seventeen percent of sexually active females and 9 percent of sexually active males did not use any contraception during their last sexual intercourse.
  - Fifty percent of sexually active males and females aged 15–19 have engaged in oral sex.
  - Ten to twenty percent of sexually active males and females aged 15–19 have engaged in anal sex with someone of the opposite sex; 3-6 percent of sexually active males aged 15–19 have engaged in anal sex with a male.
  - Approximately one in four sexually active teens contract an STI every year.
- Sexual Pressure and Sexual Assault
  - Twenty-five to 33 percent of 15–17-year olds feel pressure to have sex.

• Nearly 10 percent of high school students (12 percent of females and 6 percent of males) have been physically forced to have sexual intercourse.

Two of the most important factors that influence teenagers to become sexually active are peer pressure and the use of alcohol and/or drugs. Alcohol and drugs also make them more likely to engage in high-risk behaviors, such as unprotected sex. According to the NSFG, 23 percent of high school students who had sexual intercourse in 2005 drank alcohol or used drugs before their last sexual intercourse.

☞ Two of the most important factors that influence teenagers' decisions to become sexually active are peer pressure and the use of alcohol and/or drugs.

But, not all teens are having sex. According to the NSFG, adolescents who choose to remain virgins cited fear of pregnancy (94 percent) and fear of contracting HIV/AIDS (92 percent) as the top reasons for abstaining from vaginal intercourse. Eighty-four percent cited moral and religious reasons for abstaining from vaginal intercourse. This is an important point for parents to keep in mind if they are wondering if the HPV vaccination will promote sexual promiscuity in their children.

Sexual intercourse only forms part of the picture of adolescent sexuality. Some teens who abstain from coital (vaginal) sexual intercourse still engage in oral sex and/or anal sex. The NSFG showed that approximately 20 percent of males and females who abstained from vaginal intercourse on moral or religious grounds engaged in oral sex (Mosher et al. 2005), and a smaller percentage of them also engaged in anal sex. Teens who engage in oral and anal sex view these forms of sexual activity as more acceptable than vaginal sex, because there is almost no chance of their getting pregnant. They also believe that noncoital forms of sex are of a lesser threat to their moral and religious beliefs; unfortunately, they do not seem to realize that these acts also increase their risk for sexually transmitted infections.

Studies have shown that teenagers with involved parents are more likely to delay the initiation of sexual activity than those teenagers who do not have any parental guidance on sex-related topics such as abstinence and on the psychological and physiological side effects of sexual activity. Now, with the introduction of HPV vaccines for 11-and 12-year olds, a window of opportunity has been opened for parents and health-care providers to give some anticipatory behavioral guidance to adolescents. Besides, if you, as parents, decide to have your daughter vaccinated, you can still, by all means, without hypocrisy, inform her that this is not a green flag for her to immediately have sex; rather, it is a strong message that you care about her health. The message should not be either abstinence or sexual activity, but both. You can use HPV vaccination as an opportunity to remind her that when she does become sexually active, she *must* use protection, because although this vaccine will provide her with an additional layer of protection toward the most dangerous types of HPV infections, it will not keep her from getting pregnant or contracting other STIs. The HPV vaccine *cannot, will not,* and *should not* replace proper parenting and discussions with your children about sexuality.

WHAT PARENTS THINK ABOUT THE VACCINE AND ITS ACCEPTABILITY

Parental attitudes are crucial to the acceptance of the HPV vaccines. To date, overall parental knowledge about HPV infections and their relationship to cervical cancer and genital warts is low (Waller et al. 2003). Nearly 20 million Americans have this virus, and yet more than half to three-quarters of the women in the United States have either not heard about the virus or are not aware that HPV types cause virtually 100 percent of cervical cancers and genital warts.

Parents' acceptance is usually influenced by the attitudes of their peers and their health-care providers. Their acceptance is also high when they perceive the disease's consequence to be serious, and when they have had some personal experience with the disease themselves (Dempsey et al. 2006). On the other hand, acceptance is low among parents who have a poor disease-specific knowledge of the vaccine or who have a low concern about HPV-related diseases. In addition, parents' acceptance is low among those who feel that their child's personality, behavioral characteristics, and emotional immaturity place them at a minimal risk for initiating sexual activity and acquiring an STI in the near future.

Among parents who were both for and against the vaccine, many of them said that they would be more willing to accept the vaccine closer to the time of their child's sexual debut, rather than at age 11 or 12, which they believe to be far before the time that their child would consider having sex. Unfortunately, parents' knowledge of their adolescent child's sexual activity status is often inaccurate, and so relying on this cue to take action to vaccinate may be unrealistic and unreliable in relation to the child's need for protection. Many times, by the time parents find out that their child is sexually active, the child might have already been exposed to the virus. For example, a national survey showed that only half of the parents of sexually experienced eighth through eleventh graders were aware that their children were involved in some sort of sexual activity.

Vaccine acceptance was high among parents in the United Kingdom, Australia, and Canada. While many parents in these countries did not think that their daughters were at any risk of contracting HPV at 12 years of age, they understood the need for vaccinating at an early age. Their main concern was the long-term safety provided by the vaccine. Even among Mexican women, in whom cervical cancer rates are very high and whose knowledge about HPV and its connection to cervical cancer was very poor, acceptance for the vaccine was high once they were educated on the subject. A recent study found that educational interventions increased parental support for the vaccine from 55 to 75 percent (Gust et al. 2006). Needless to say, the most frequently mentioned reason for parents to accept the vaccines was the simple desire to protect their child from the disease.

The key to success for any public health measure is to gain community acceptance. Social and cultural acceptance will play a very important role in the introduction of the HPV vaccines in the developing world. Perhaps the lessons learned from the implementation of the vaccines there will help us iron out the obstacles among various religious and ethnic groups in our own country.

> ☞ The key to success for any public health measure is to gain community acceptability.

REVISITING OTHER REASONS TO BE VACCINATED

There is only one vaccine that is currently available in the United States, *Gardasil,* which covers HPV types 6 and 11—the types that cause 90 percent of genital warts—and HPV types 16 and 18—which cause 70 percent of cervical cancers. The other vaccine, *Cervarix,* protects against types 16 and 18, but it has not yet been approved in the United States. *Gardasil* is marketed as a cancer vaccine because its primary focus at this time is for prevention of cervical cancer. But knowing that the statistics for cervical cancer are very low in this country, and assuming, for a moment, that our daughters will be getting their gynecological exams and Pap tests on a scheduled basis for early detection of cervical cancer, are there any other compelling reasons to administer the vaccines to them? Personally, I believe the following reasons are more applicable for most girls and women in the United States, even if they have chosen not to be sexually active before marriage and will only have a monogamous relationship after marriage. These may also be the reasons for girls and young women in other developed countries, where the rates of cervical cancer are low, to consider getting the vaccine.

Sexual Assault

For some girls and women, sexual activity could occur against their will, through rape, incest, or other forms of sexual assault. Though no parent would ever want to imagine that a daughter might be a victim of sexual assault, it is, unfortunately, one of the unwelcome realities of life. Around 12 percent of female high school students are assaulted every year in the United States. Though the vaccines do not give protection against other STIs, they can at least protect against those types that cause most cervical cancers. *Gardasil* also gives protection against 90 percent of genital warts.

History of Partner

One thing is clear: having sex once or having only one partner does *not* mean one is not at risk. Very few women can say with absolute certainly that their partners did not have sexual contact with anyone else prior to their meeting.

Emotional Upheaval

One cannot minimize the emotional upheaval that HPV can cause. As HPV is mostly acquired by the 15–24-year-old age groups, the emotional impact of carrying a virus that can lie dormant in the body indefinitely and for which there is no cure can be daunting. Therefore, the vaccine can be of benefit in relieving this potential anxiety. (Refer to Chapter 5 for an in-depth coverage of emotional aspects of HPV.)

Genital Warts

There are over a million cases of genital warts each year in the United States. Genital warts are unsightly, uncomfortable, and recurrent, and they require several treatments and visits to the clinic or doctor's office. They cause psychological trauma, and much time, energy, and money is spent on treating them. Nearly $200 million is spent annually on the treatment of genital warts in this country. Ninety percent of genital warts are caused by HPV 6 and 11. *Gardasil* has demonstrated nearly 100 percent effectiveness preventing warts caused by HPV 6 and 11 in the absence of prior exposure to those types. *Cervarix* (the other HPV vaccine awaiting approval in the United States) does not cover the types that cause genital warts.

Cervical Dysplasias

As discussed in earlier chapters, cervical dysplasia is a condition where abnormal cells are present in the cervix. Most cervical dysplasias resolve on their own; some, if not treated, progress to invasive cancer. Cervical dysplasia may require follow-up procedures and testing and several visits to your health-care facility. Both vaccines, *Gardasil* and *Cervarix,* have been shown to offer 98–100 percent protection in preventing CIN II/CIN III (precursors of invasive cervical cancer) caused by HPV types 16 and 18. This may mean fewer cases of abnormal Pap tests in the future and, subsequently, fewer follow-ups and procedures.

It should be noted that the above reasons in *no way* undermine the importance of the vaccines in reducing the rates of cervical cancer.

Obviously, if our daughters do not get Pap smears or other tests recommended in the future for detecting early cervical cancer, then the vaccine will be of tremendous benefit in giving them protection against 70 percent of cervical cancers. This will undoubtedly reduce the rates of invasive cervical cancer both in this country and around the world, assuming that they work just as well in the real-world scenario as they have in clinical trials.

So, for parents who are convinced that the HPV vaccines may have benefits outside of preventing cervical cancer alone, but still fear the effect on their teenagers' sexual behavior, it may be worth mentioning the following important point again: there are negative consequences of sexual behavior, such as the threat of pregnancy and AIDS, that are far more immediate than the threat of cancer in teenagers' minds. Besides, the vaccine only protects against a few strains of HPV, and not against all sexually transmitted diseases. Therefore, there is no reason the protection against cervical cancer afforded by the vaccines would lead young teens to become sexually promiscuous. Paramount emphasis and priority should still be placed on teaching teens to follow healthy and safe lifestyles.

STI versus Cancer Vaccine

The vaccine is marketed as a cancer vaccine in the United States. As we all know, the "C" word instills a tremendous amount of fear in most of us. But the good news is that cervical cancer is rare in this country. According to the ACS, cervical cancer accounts for only 0.6 percent of all cancer deaths per year in the United States. Even though one would not like to lose a single life to cervical cancer, in comparison, the incidence and costs of treating genital warts and cervical dysplasias are nearly 10 times more than that of treating cervical cancer. So should the vaccine be promoted as a cancer prevention vaccine, or should we paint a more accurate picture and promote it as both a cancer and an STI vaccine? After all, cervical cancer is a sexually transmitted disease.

When a disease is described as sexually transmitted, it is tempting to immediately assume that it only afflicts the promiscuous. This is a dangerous attitude, as what is and is not "promiscuous" are obviously relative and a matter of opinion. "Promiscuous is anyone who has had one more sexual partner than you!" was a favorite saying of one of my professors during my training in Obstetrics and Gynecology.

It is clear from opinion polls that the vaccine has considerably higher acceptance (63 percent approval rating) when marketed as a cancer vaccine versus an STI vaccine (43 percent approval rating). Also, it is quite normal for us to be wary of an STI vaccine, as encouraging our daughters to get it could almost seem like an admission that they are engaging in risky sexual behavior—a label that no parents would like to see applied to their daughters. The question, then, is how do we present the vaccine so that the ultimate objectives are still met, while safeguarding the lives of teenagers? Whereas the pharmaceutical companies that manufacture the vaccine have to face myriads of objections to marketing it as a STI vaccine, I as a physician and a health educator have the privilege of presenting the vaccine as I see and believe it when considering the public's best interest.

Public education makes vaccine acceptance easier. For example, I was recently talking about the vaccine with a 22-year-old patient of mine who was in a serious relationship and was contemplating being sexually active. "I don't think I need the vaccine, because I am very health conscious and will always get my Pap tests," she said to me. However, when I told her about the other potential advantages of the vaccines, she immediately told me, "Now, I think I may be better off getting the vaccine anyway. These reasons that you mentioned outside of the prevention of cervical cancer made more sense to me in my case." The moral of this story again highlights the importance of awareness and education; if the public is educated, and the HPV vaccines perform as promised in the real world, it will not be easy to ignore the positive impact that they can have on HPV-related diseases, even though HPV is a sexually transmitted disease.

WEIGHING THE PROS AND CONS

This section of the chapter serves as a review of topics that have already been discussed in detail in various chapters of the book. The intent is to provide a quick reference of the merits and demerits of the vaccine.

Pros of the Vaccine

Saves Lives by Preventing Cervical Cancer

- There are nearly 11,000 cases of cervical cancer per year in the United States, with 4,000 deaths attributed to it annually.
- Globally, there are around 500,000 cases of cervical cancer annually, with 250,000 deaths directly related to them.
- The vaccine is 98–100 percent effective in preventing cervical cancer caused by HPV 16 and 18, the types that account for 70 percent of all cervical cancers.

Minimizes the Occurrence of Genital Warts

- There are around 1 million cases of genital warts per year in the United States, with both men and women equally affected.
- *Gardasil* is the only vaccine that is almost 100 percent effective HPV types 6 and 11, which account for 90 percent of genital warts.

Reduces Precancerous Diagnoses

Cervical Dysplasias—CIN I and CIN II/III
The vaccine prevents the development of CIN I and CIN II/III caused by HPV 16 and 18, and decreases the number of procedures such as colposcopy, cervical biopsy, and LEEP used for diagnosis and treatment of cervical dysplasias. (Refer to Chapter 4 for more details on HPV-related precancerous and cancerous lesions.)

Vulvar Intraepithelial Neoplasia (VIN) Grade 2 and Grade 3
VIN refers to the presence of abnormal squamous cells in the vulva, which can progress to cancer if not treated in a timely fashion. According to National Cancer Institute estimates, there were 3,490 new cases of vulvar cancers and 880 deaths from it in the United States in 2007. The good news is that nearly 50 percent of VIN grades 2 and 3 (precancerous lesions) are caused by HPV 16 and 18, and, the vaccines are 98–100 percent effective against these types.

Vaginal Intraepithelial Neoplasia (VAIN) Grade 2 and Grade 3
Like VIN, VAIN refers to the presence of abnormal squamous cells in the vagina, which can progress to cancer if left untreated. According to the National Cancer Institute estimates, there were about 2,140 new cases of vaginal cancer and 790 deaths in the United States in the year 2007. Nearly 50 percent of VAIN grades 2 and 3 (precancerous lesions) are caused by HPV 16 and 18, for which the vaccines are very effective.

Cervical Adenocarcinoma in situ *(AIS)*
The majority of cervical dysplasias occur in the squamous epithelium. The rest occur in the glandular epithelium. AIS occurs when the abnormal cells of the glandular epithelium have not yet broken through the basement membrane and have not invaded the adjacent tissues. HPV 18 is the dominant virus in AIS. The vaccines are 98–100 percent effective against HPV 18.

Minimizes Emotional Consequences Related to an STI

- The emotional consequences of having a virus that is sexually transmitted for which there is no cure can be substantial for most.
- The vaccine can help alleviate some of these concerns by offering protection against their targeted strains respectively.

Facilitates Sex Education

Parents can use the HPV vaccine to initiate discussions on teen sexuality in preadolescent and adolescent girls. If the vaccine is introduced for boys and men in the near future, it will ease discussions of sex education with them, too.

Offers Other Potential Benefits

Cross-Protection
Cervarix, the vaccine awaiting FDA approval in the United States, has shown significant protection against HPV types 45, 31, and 52. HPV types 45 and 31 are the third and fourth most common causes of cervical cancer. Recent data has shown that *Gardasil* may also provide cross-protection against 10 additional cancer-causing HPV strains not targeted by the vaccine.

Recurrent Respiratory Papillomas
Gardasil, the vaccine that covers HPV types 6 and 11, may also prove to protect against respiratory papillomas—benign growths in the airway tract.

Oral Cancer
According to the American Cancer Society, HPV may be responsible for about 20 to 30 percent of the estimated 34,360 cases of the cancers of the mouth and throat (oropharyngeal cancers). HPV-related throat cancer strikes about 11,000 new men and women each year. Most of them are caused by HPV 16. The vaccine could prove beneficial in preventing HPV 16 and 18 related oral cancers.

Anal Cancer
The American Cancer Society estimates that in 2007, about 4,650 new cases of anal cancer will be diagnosed in the United States, out of which 2,750 will occur in women and 1,900 will occur in men. An estimated 430 women and 260 men will die from it, totalling 690 in 2007. Ninety percent of anal cancers are caused by HPV 16 and 18, with HPV 16 causing the majority of them. Phase 3 clinical trials have shown that *Gardasil* results in a 100 percent reduction in the incidence of HPV-associated anogenital diseases in young women.

Cons of the Vaccine

As is the case with most new vaccines, the HPV vaccines raise many questions related to duration of immunity, long-term side effects, and their true effectiveness in preventing cervical cancer in the real world. Other barriers are the inconvenience of requiring three shots at specified time intervals, high purchase costs, and the demographics of targeted patients.

Pain at the Injection Site

Pain is the most common side effect. Eight out of 10 women report pain at the injection site after vaccination. This pain is usually mild and resolves itself in 24–48 hours.

Severe Allergy to Yeast

Gardasil should not be administered to those who have a severe allergy to yeast. *Cervarix* may be a better choice as this vaccine is not grown on yeast.

Age of Vaccination

Many parents feel that the age (11–12 years) is too young to be vaccinated against a sexually transmitted disease. Also, some argue that the vaccine was tested in the 16–24 year age group as opposed to the age group for which it is recommended. Based on the statistics of teen sex, it makes sense to vaccinate all girls at 11–12 years of age. However, for those who are uncomfortable with this, the vaccine can be administered up to 26 years of age. Keep in mind that the vaccine is most effective when administered before a patient is exposed to the targeted virus—which in this case means it is most effective when administered before initiation of ANY sexual activity.

Duration of Immunity

The duration of vaccine protection is unclear. So far, the vaccine has been found to be effective for at least 5 years without any proof of waning immunity during this time period. This information will be updated periodically as additional data become available.

Promotion of Early Sexual Activity

One commonly voiced objection among those opposed to the vaccine is that the vaccine has to be administered before sexual debut. Some believe that this will encourage early sexual activity as the vaccine's purpose will necessitate teaching girls about sex instead of "abstinence only" until marriage (Davis et al. 2004; Olshen et al. 2005). I believe that there are at least three main reasons

> ☞ The vaccines do not protect against all STIs. Therefore, they will not promote sexual promiscuity among teenagers as other precautions will have to be taken.

why the vaccines will not promote early sexual activity. First, it is not a vaccine for *all* STIs. Second, we now know that teens do not abstain from sex for the fear of acquiring a sexually transmitted disease other than HIV/AIDS. Finally, the vaccine does not prevent pregnancy, one of the major reasons teens abstain from sex. Therefore, vaccinating against HPV should not increase teen sexual activity.

Narrow Range of Coverage

There are more than a dozen types of HPV that can cause cancer. Neither of the vaccines covers all of the cancer-causing types.

Not a Treatment

The vaccine has no therapeutic effect on HPV-related diseases. As a result, if a girl or a woman receives the vaccine after she has already been exposed to the vaccine-targeted strains, the vaccine will not prevent diseases from those types. Studies are underway in developing preventive *cum* therapeutic vaccines.

Multiple Doses

Three doses of the vaccine are required to acquire full benefits from the vaccination. This can lead to compliance issues that are usually associated with multiple dosing schedules.

Will Not Replace Cervical Screening

The vaccine only targets two of the cancer-causing strains. Therefore, Pap smears and/or HPV DNA testing will have to be continued according to the American Cancer Society protocol. The vaccine should not give a false sense of security that it is a replacement for other preventive strategies.

Cost of the Vaccine

At $360 for a series of three shots, the vaccine is not affordable for many and certainly not for those women who will benefit from it the most. Work is in progress to provide better coverage to the underprivileged and the uninsured.

Long-Term Effects

Another concern for parents is the possible long-term effects of the vaccine. With the increasing number of immunizations that children are getting these days, parents worry that there might be some long-term insidious effects such as allergies, arthritis, and autoimmune disease. In an autoimmune disease, the body attacks itself. In the case of the vaccines, there is the potential possibility that the high titers of antibody response that they evoke could attack some other part of the body that is chemically related to the vaccine. This has not been proven to be the case so far.

Not Approved in Men

HPV is a sexually transmitted disease, but the vaccine has not been approved for men in the United States. The vaccine would have a direct health benefit in men in preventing genital warts, as well as oral, anal, and penile cancers. There would also be an indirect benefit to women through vaccinating men, as it would help decrease the spread of HPV to them. Studies are still in progress, and results should be available in

Table 9.1 Vaccine Pros and Cons Overview

Vaccine pros	Vaccine cons
Prevents 70% of cervical cancers	Often causes pain at the injection site
Prevents 90% of genital warts (*Gardasil* only)	Cannot be administered to patients with severe yeast allergy (only *Gardasil*)
Prevents 35%– 70% of cervical dyspalsias	Age of vaccination is too young
Prevents approximately 50% of vulvar dysplasias	Duration of immunity is not completely known
Prevents approximately 50% of vaginal dysplasias	Safety profile and long-term effects are still under study
Prevents approximately 70% of adenocarcinoma *in situ* of the cervix.	Is only a preventive vaccine— no therapeutic effect
Minimizes the upheaval of carrying a STI for which there is no cure	Requires multiple dosing
Encourages sex education in preadolescents	Will not replace Pap tests or HPV DNA testing
Has cross-protection with a few other cancer-causing HPVs.	Has a high purchase price
Has the potential to prevent 30% of HPV-related oropharyngeal cancers.	Not approved in men
Has the potential to prevent 70%–90% of anal dysplasias and anal cancer in men and women.	May promote sexual promiscuity according to some

the next couple of years. (Refer to Chapter 7 for more details on vaccine for men.)

The pros and cons of the vaccines are summarized in Table 9.1.

Compelling Issues That Parents Have with Vaccines That Doctors Do Not Discuss

Oftentimes, parents have many questions about topics surrounding vaccines, but, unfortunately, they do not find the opportunity to review these issues with their health-care providers. In order to give a more comprehensive overview of the vaccine, I have included a set of compelling issues that I hope will benefit those parents who are still have questions and concerns about the merit of the vaccine.

Vaccines and Autism

The news story in March 2008 of compensation awarded for vaccine-related symptoms of autism has created many headlines and has many parents worried about the relationship between vaccines and autism. Controversy has existed over whether a mercury-containing preservative in vaccines called thiomerosal can cause autism in children. Even though neither of the HPV vaccines contains thiomerosal, the issue is compelling enough to require special mention.

Autism is a complex developmental disability that typically appears during the first three to five years of life and affects the area of the brain that is responsible for social interaction and communication skills. Children with autism lack eye contact and have repetitive behaviors. Research continues to show that there is no link between thiomerosal and autism (Sugarman 2007). In fact, a study published in *Journal Watch Pediatrics and Adolescent Medicine* in January 2008 showed that, in spite of the removal of thiomerosal from all the vaccines for children under six years old since 2003 (with the exception of some influenza vaccines), the prevalence of autism in children has actually increased. Experts are now looking to see if genetics and environmental factors have a role to play. The good news is that the HPV vaccine does not contain thiomerosal, and the earliest it can be given is at nine years of age—well past the age when autism typically appears.

Vaccines and Seizures

Some believe that the aluminum salts contained in vaccines are responsible for brain diseases such as seizures and Alzheimer's dementia. Aluminum is an element found in trace amounts in several products in nature, including foods and vaccines. Most vaccines contain traces of aluminum to promote antibody production. Both of the HPV vaccines contain aluminum. The compound in *Cervarix* has a unique structure that is said to prolong the duration of immunity of the vaccine. According to the National Cancer Institute and the Alzheimer's Society, there seems to be no direct link between aluminum contained in vaccines and brain damage.

Skepticism over FDA Approvals

Some parents are skeptical about the FDA's approval of vaccines. The classic example of a cause for this skepticism is the Rotavirus vaccine that was introduced in August 1998 under the name *Rotashield*. Rotavirus is the most common virus that causes diarrhea and dehydration in infants. *Rotashield* was an oral vaccine that was genetically engineered from the live rotavirus. However, in August 1999, after administering 1 million doses to infants across the country, the CDC pulled the vaccine from the market because an increased number of cases of a serious bowel disease called intussusception was reported after the administration of the vaccine.

The HPV vaccine *Gardasil* has been on the market since June 2006. As of April 30, 2008, over 12 million doses of the vaccine have been distributed, but it is not known how many doses have actually been administered. So far, serious adverse reactions from *Gardasil* have been low. Fifteen deaths have been reported in patients who have had the *Gardasil* vaccination, but according to the CDC, the reported deaths in vaccine recipients do not appear to be causally related to the HPV vaccine. The CDC is continuing to monitor these events. (Refer to Chapter 6 for more details of vaccine-related adverse effects.)

Reporting of Drug Trials

Consumers who are already wary of vaccines have one more reason to stand by their convictions. Recent data showed that in the case of some of the popular antidepressants such as Prozac and Paxil, the pharmaceutical companies, in order to win the government's approval, only published data that had favorable outcomes, while hiding the unfavorable results. These trials were done in the years 1987–2004. In order to rectify this problem, Congress passed legislation in 2007 that requires more transparency into all clinical trials.

The HPV vaccine *Gardasil* was approved in June 2006 for commercial use. We can only hope that we are working with the most reliable data available. So far, over 30,000 women have been tested worldwide with each of the vaccines, and both have undergone extensive and advanced phase 3 clinical trials. Invasive cervical cancer typically follows a slowly progressive course that can be prevented at various stages. Both vaccines have shown to prevent these precursor stages (CIN II and CIN III), but we do not have proof that they actually prevent the cancer from developing. As such, until the real effectiveness of the vaccine is known (which will take decades) there is a leap of faith involved in its science.

Worries over "Replacement Disease"

Some fear that with the introduction of the HPV vaccines, HPV strains not covered by the vaccine might step up and find the perfect ecological niche to thrive and cause disease. This phenomenon, called the "replacement disease," was seen with the pneumococcal vaccine *Prevnar*, which was introduced in the United States in 2000. *Prevnar* was introduced to reduce the number of cases of pneumococcal-associated respiratory tract diseases in infants and children. But, at the same time, reports showed an increase in the number of cases of respiratory diseases caused by the pneumococcal strains not covered by the vaccine (replacement disease). However, the overall impact in the increase of these non-vaccine–covered cases was negligible when compared to the substantial reduction in the number of respiratory cases due to *Prevnar* (Albrich 2007). Certainly, such a phenomenon is possible with the HPV vaccine. In fact, there are a few reports that already allude to the emergence of non-vaccine–covered types of HPV, but so far they have not been of any clinical significance.

Scare from the Failed Merck's AIDS Vaccine

In the Fall of 2007, there was a catastrophic setback to the development of Merck's much anticipated AIDS vaccine. Merck discontinued its trials when results showed that some vaccine recipients actually developed HIV infections after receiving the vaccine. The AIDS vaccine was genetically engineered to deliver three synthetic HIV genes through a disabled cold virus, none of which could reproduce to cause AIDS or colds. The scientists do not believe that the vaccine was responsible for the increased number of infections, as there were other factors that came into play. Even though the details of the results are beyond the scope of this book, as far as the HPV vaccines are concerned, neither of the vaccines has any viral genes, synthetic or natural, and there are no cold viruses engineered into the vaccines, either.

Which Is Better—Natural or Vaccine-induced Immunity?

Unfortunately, there is no simple answer to this question. Natural immunity to a particular disease is acquired when a person is exposed to the specific organism that causes the disease. Obviously, this would involve considerable risk—for example, in order to gain a natural immunity from polio, one would become paralyzed in the process. On the other hand, immunity acquired from the vaccine causes a person to produce antibodies without developing the actual disease in almost all cases. It has also been found that, in the case of the HPV vaccines, the antibody titers produced by the vaccines for the targeted strains are nearly 10-fold higher than antibody titers produced by natural infections. At the present time, it is clear neither if this heightened immunity leads to that much higher and longer effectiveness nor if the lower levels of antibody titers produced by natural HPV infections are adequate enough to protect against future infections from the same HPV types.

In either case, having a robust immunity that stems from regular exercise, a well-balanced diet, stress reduction strategies, and an overall healthy lifestyle is essential to keep all infections at bay.

Personal History

Every child is an individual human being, with a unique medical history and set of genes that may explain why some children react adversely to vaccines while others do not. Even though there is no scientific evidence to prove that genetic variations are responsible for some of the deleterious effects of vaccines, common sense dictates that you should discuss any of your concerns with your doctor before deciding to vaccinate.

What Are the Main Differences between the Two HPV Vaccines?

The two main HPV vaccines are *Gardasil* by Merck and *Cervarix* by GlaxoSmithKline (GSK). *Gardasil* protects against four strains of HPV, namely 6, 11, 16, and 18 (types 6 and 11 are responsible for 90 percent of genital warts and types 16 and 18 cause 70 percent of cervical cancers). *Cervarix* guards against only types 16 and 18. Therefore, *Cervarix* will not be beneficial in protecting against genital warts. In their clinical trials, GSK found *Cervarix* to provide good cross-protection against HPV types 45 and 31, which are the third and fourth most common types causing cervical cancer. In addition, a new type of adjuvant (a substance that has been added to the vaccine to enhance its effect) is being used in *Cervarix,* which according to GSK will help sustain robust and prolonged antibody titers. Whether all this will translate to superior protection against cervical cancer is not yet known. *Gardasil* is already approved in the United States, while *Cervarix* is currently awaiting FDA approval. (Refer to Table 6.1 in Chapter 6 for other differences between *Gardasil* and *Cervarix*.)

Who Really Needs the Vaccine?

As we discussed earlier, all girls between the ages of 11 and 12 can benefit from the vaccine—even those among the privileged class in whom cervical cancer rates are low as a result of better access to regular gynecological exams and Pap tests. The vaccine offers an excellent opportunity for primary prevention (prevention of development) of many lesions caused by HPV types 6, 11, 16, and 18 (*Gardasil*). This, in turn, could reduce the number of cases of genital warts and cervical dysplasias and bring down the cost and inconvenience of treating them (Elbasha et al 2007). The vaccine has the potential to offer maximum lifesaving benefits to young girls in the lower socioeconomic group in this country and the rest of the world. This is the group that either has no easy access or cannot afford the Pap test. Ironically, this is the group that has historically experienced high rates of cervical cancer and can least afford the high cost of the vaccine.

SHOULD THE VACCINE BE MANDATED—AND WILL IT?

Mandates are introduced to protect public health. The underlying principle behind mandates is that vaccinating the majority will protect the relatively few who are at high risk for acquiring the disease through induced herd immunity. Several states are considering the option to require the vaccine (see Table 1.1 in Chapter 1). Mandates have advantages, including their ability to help bridge the economic, racial, and ethnic differences between people. Mandates that require students to be vaccinated in order to go to school serve as an effective way to provide (required) access to all, regardless of socioeconomic status. In addition, requiring all children to be vaccinated at age 11–12 rather than later in life has shown to be the best way to protect a future generation of women in poor and disadvantaged areas from cervical cancer. A much higher percentage of teens in poor areas drop out of high school and engage in high-risk behaviors, thus rendering a mandate in the high school population less effective than one at a younger age, when all children are guaranteed to still be in school. It has been repeatedly shown that mass scale programs such as school mandates result in widespread coverage, and these programs surpass the traditional methods of persuasion such as education by peers, individuals, or health-care professionals. Smallpox and polio vaccines would not have had the success they did had they not been mandated. Therefore, the premise for the HPV vaccine mandate is that large-scale immunization will be the most efficient way to ensure that underprivileged girls are protected. Discounts can also be negotiated with vaccine manufacturers for mass vaccination programs.

However, when legislation was introduced to mandate the HPV vaccine in more that 20 states, within one year of its introduction to the market, the proposition backfired. Even parents who were generally not skeptics of mandates argued that unlike measles and mumps, HPV could not be spread through casual respiratory contact in a school setting. In addition, some parents believe that the vaccine undermines their authority and gives license for children to engage in sexual activity at an earlier age than they would have otherwise opted to. Many parents also had safety and ethical concerns and voiced that the "one size fits all" approach to the HPV vaccine was inappropriate, and that it was the government's job to provide the science, and the individual's right to choose whether or not to utilize it. Finally, because the risk of cervical cancer is relatively small in the United States, some parents argued that mandating the HPV vaccine is less about safeguarding the public as a whole and more about the government intruding into people's personal lives to strip them of their autonomy.

Vaccine mandates vary from state to state. The controversy over the HPV vaccine mandates has so far prevented them from being adopted in any state so far. The Virginia legislature passed a school vaccine requirement in 2007 with a liberal opt-out clause made available. However, it is currently (2008) considering a bill that would delay the vaccine requirement.

Opt-out clauses are put in place to mitigate the effects of governmental intrusion. They allow parents to exempt their children from vaccination requirements for medical reasons. In 48 states, parents can opt out of immunizations for religious reasons, and, in 20 states, parents can opt out on philosophical grounds beyond religious and medical reasons.

Although there are advantages to leaving the decision to mandate in the hands of the states rather than in the hands of a federal organization, it creates a confusing pattern of rules and regulations that adds difficulty in developing a clear and uniform set of guidelines nationwide. In addition, one has to be really careful about exercising their rights to opt out, as it can undermine the underlying mandate principle and defeat the whole purpose of minimizing the public health risk.

Making the decision to mandate the HPV vaccine is a major undertaking, and it requires a great measure of patience. After all, a recommendation is being made for a whole generation of American children for a disease that will not be apparent for the next several decades. In my opinion, in order to mandate the HPV vaccine, the following categories should be fully addressed.

Public Education

The public's knowledge of HPV is poor. Therefore, the public must be educated about HPV infections and the potential benefits of the vaccine before putting mandates in place. Parents should also be informed that the vaccine is not a substitute for routine Pap tests, as the vaccine does not cover all HPV types that cause cervical cancer.

In addition, as African Americans and Hispanics are at the highest rate for getting cervical cancer, these groups should be targeted aggressively. Schools with high enrollment of ethnic minorities should receive adequate funding in order to achieve high levels of coverage.

Clinical Experience

As time goes by, additional data about the side effects and efficacy of the vaccines will become apparent. But without having adequate information, mandating the vaccine at this time is a premature move. Both of the vaccine makers should continue to follow participants from the vaccine trials to learn more about the long-term safety and efficacy of HPV vaccines.

Duration of Immunity

The duration of immunity for the HPV vaccines has still not been established. So far, the vaccine has been found to be effective for at least five years. Therefore, there is no proof that booster shots will not be required in the future. Thus, whoever is covering the costs of the vaccine—whether it is individuals, private insurance companies, or the government—should take into consideration that booster shots may be required at a future date. If not, the mandate would be futile and would defeat the purpose of vaccinating girls at 11–12 years of age, only to find out that at 17, the time when they need it the most, the protective effect of the vaccine has been greatly diminished or has entirely vanished.

Allocation of Funds

Next, there is the question of cost: who is going to pay for the mandated vaccine and how—at what expense and the trading of which public funding? Time should be given to state public health agencies to allocate funds and negotiate with vaccine makers for discounted prices. In addition, innovative funding strategies should be developed to ensure adequate vaccine supply and delivery to populations with the highest mortality from the devastating disease.

Vaccine Injury Compensation

Another issue that needs attention is how vaccine victims would be compensated if an injury occurred. When a vaccine is mandated by the state, the state has to bear the brunt of the compensation and not the vaccine maker.

Cost-Effectiveness

Is it worth spending money to immunize 2 million girls every year in the 11–12-year-old range in order to prevent 10,000 cases of cervical cancer? Studies have been conducted to show that the cost-effectiveness of the vaccine in preventing HPV 16 and 18 diseases is substantial, in spite of continuing current cervical screening programs. This does not take into account the fact that the vaccine *Gardasil* can prevent 90 percent of genital warts, in which case the cost-effectiveness would be even greater. It seems that, in the long run, the vaccine can save significant amounts of health-care dollars now spent toward treating HPV infections.

Vaccine in Men

Studies have shown that the prevalence of HPV infections in men is as high as it is in women, and that men are likely to transmit the virus to their partners. Therefore, if the underlying principle of immunizations is to vaccinate the masses for the good of the few, one can argue that it is unfair and unjust to put all the focus on women when, in actuality, HPV is sexually transmitted, and men should be equally responsible for preventing its transmission. Until more information is obtained about the vaccine in males, it would be unethical to compel only girls to get the vaccine in order to attend publicly funded schools.

There are two issues that have to be clarified and resolved before mandating the vaccine; first, a longer-term safety profile has to be known, and, second, the issue of the vaccines in men has to be clarified. Till then, I am afraid the choice to vaccinate should be left to individuals and not to the states. The vaccine should be offered on a voluntary basis as a part of a comprehensive package that is aimed at preventing cervical cancer and other consequences of HPV infections.

Should You Vaccinate Your Daughter?

Is this not the main reason you have been reading this book—to arrive at this very point where you have to make the BIG decision with clarity of thought and your purpose clearly defined? For those who have come this far and made up your mind, congratulations are in order. However, for those of you who still have a few uneasy doubts lingering, I have just a few more thoughts to share with you.

Here Is My Thought Process

- HPV, a sexually transmitted infection that causes genital warts and cervical cancer, is a highly prevalent virus in sexually active men and women.
- Over 50 percent of girls are sexually active by the time they graduate from high school. Parents may not always know when their children become sexually active.
- Cervical cancer is rare in this country; a well-established Pap testing program has significantly reduced the rates of cervical cancer. Despite this, cervical cancer has not been eradicated. Therefore, if administered *before* sexual debut the vaccine would provide an added layer of nearly 100 percent protection against HPV types 16 and 18 that cause a vast majority of cervical cancers.
- The importance of HPV cannot be based on its reference to cervical cancer only. Genital warts are a common HPV disease manifestation. Genital warts are unsightly and uncomfortable and require recurrent treatment. *Gardasil* can confer 100 percent protection against almost all genital warts caused by HPV types 6 and 11.
- The HPV vaccine would also prevent the majority of cervical dysplasias and minimize the follow-ups and procedures required for managing such lesions—prevention is better than treatment or cure.
- The emotional turmoil of having an incurable STI can play havoc in the minds of women, particularly young women. The HPV vaccine can mitigate this to a great extent.
- Finally, the short-term benefits of the vaccines are just as important as the long-term benefits. Therefore, it is worth vaccinating girls and young women to reduce the physical, psycho-social, and economic burden of HPV infections.

> ☞ **Vaccination, along with regular gynecological exams and cervical screening, will offer women the best possible protection against both the short- and long-term consequences of HPV infections.**

Patient Education

Patient education is crucial in reducing the physical, mental, and economic burden related to HPV infections and cervical cancers. According to a survey published in the *Journal of Obstetrics and Gynecology*, the current knowledge of HPV among inner-city high school students is unacceptably low. Nearly 87 percent of students had not heard about HPV. Even among women who attended well-women clinics, only a third had heard about HPV. Strangely enough, in those who had abnormal Pap smears and underwent colposcopy, the knowledge of HPV was lower when compared to other sexually transmitted diseases.

It is clear the vaccine program can only be successful if there is a coordinated effort among patients, parents, health professionals, drug companies, and policy-makers for its implementation. Patient education, removal of societal barriers, and effective distribution of the vaccines are key to improving immunization rates.

With the advances in genetic engineering and immunobiology, the development of vaccines against other STIs such as chlamydia, herpes simplex, and HIV are more promising than ever before. Most of these vaccines are presumed to target adolescents—the population that is at the highest risk of contracting these diseases. Because science evolves at a much more rapid pace than human nature, I am sure we will yet again find ourselves at the crossroads of science, religion, technology, and politics.

We parents want to do what is best for our children. We want them to enjoy the best quality of life possible and protect them from as many diseases as we can. We can only hope that they make the right decisions when they leave the protective cocoon of their homes. Vaccines can save millions of lives, but at times they may harm a few along the way. The line between these two may seem fine and hard to tread at times, but it is a line that we must clearly define, particularly when so many lives of the future generation—our children—are at stake.

KEY FACTS

- The HPV vaccine will not—and more importantly, should not—replace parental guidance to children on sex education and awareness.
- The vaccine is preventive, not therapeutic. Therefore, it works best if administered before sexual debut.
- The vaccines will not promote sexual promiscuity.
- The vaccine does not protect against other STIs; therefore standard precautions still have to be taken.
- The vaccine is not mandated by any state at this time.
- Complete details on safety issues and duration of immunity are not yet fully known.
- Public education is key to vaccine acceptability and should be an integral part of the vaccination process.

10

Vaccines on the Global Front: Unique Challenges and Opportunities

Myth: The lack of adequate treatment options is the main cause for the higher rates of cervical cancer in the developing world.

Fact: Poor political will and lack of awareness that cervical cancer is a preventable public health problem are the main causes for the higher rates of cervical cancer in the developing world.

Cervical cancer is a preventable public health problem. As Dr. Connie Trimble, Director of the Cervical Cancer Dysplasia Center at Johns Hopkins School of Medicine thoughtfully said, "Here's a cancer where we know the cause, we know how to screen for it, we know how to treat it early, and it's still the second-leading cancer of women worldwide." Every year in the regions of Latin America, North America, and South America, close to 100,000 cases of cervical cancer occur, with nearly 38,000 resulting in death. Subregional differences exist, with mortality rates from cervical cancer being four or five times higher in Latin America and the Caribbean than in North America. The disparity in the number of cervical cancer cases in different communities is not due to genetic or biological differences; rather, it is attributable to socioeconomic inequalities. Higher rates of cervical cancer are closely associated with lack of financial resources, low educational levels, and poor health-care facilities. In addition, poorly organized outreach programs, suboptimal professional training, and inadequate political support have made the implementation of a public health solution to cervical cancer in developing nations a formidable task. There are more than 470,000 new cases of cervical cancer and 233,000 deaths from it each year worldwide.

Table 10.1 Number of Incident Cases and Deaths from Cervical Cancer Worldwide—Statistics from 2002

Regions	Number of cases per year	Number of deaths per year
World	492,800	273,200
More developed	83,400	39,500
Less developed	409,400	233,700
North America	14,600	4,600
United States	13,000	4,100
Central and South America	65,400	29,500
Africa	78,700	61,300
Asia	265,700	142,600
Europe	59,700	29,600
Australia	682	227
Caribbean	6,300	3,100

Source: Based on information obtained from the International Agency for Research on Cancer.

Table 10.1 shows the occurrence of cervical cancer and resulting deaths in different regions of the world in 2002. From this table, one can see that the total number of new cervical cases around the world is about 493,000 cases per year out of which 273,000 result in deaths (Sankaranarayanan 2006). Out of this, nearly 85 percent of the burden (410,000 cases and 233,000 deaths) occurs in the developing world in areas such as Latin America, Asia, and Africa. The remaining 83,000 cases and 40,000 deaths occur in the more developed countries such as the United States, the United Kingdom, and Canada. What is disappointing here is that, even though the number of cases of cervical cancer in the developed world is far fewer than the number of cases in the developing world, the ratio for cervical cancer cases to cervical cancer deaths in both developed and developing countries is nearly the same. These data possibly show that affluent and industrialized nations are as delinquent in reaching out to the socioeconomically disadvantaged segments of the population as developing countries are. These statistics are quite disturbing as they reveal much work needs to be done all over the world to reduce the ravages caused by cervical cancer.

☞ Cervical cancer is a preventable public health problem.

The biggest success in the more developed world in controlling cervical cancer cases has been achieved with the implementation of widespread screening programs, such as Pap tests, to detect precancerous lesions before they progress to invasive cancer. As we discussed earlier, the Pap test has transformed cervical cancer from being the leading killer of women in the United States about 50 years ago to the 12th ranking cause of death today. Currently, about 11,000 new cases and nearly 4,000 deaths from cervical cancer occur annually in the United States.

Against this backdrop, it is important to understand some of the barriers that developing nations face, as well as the challenges they will face in the introduction of the vaccine, and the important steps that are necessary to take to contribute to the global prevention of cervical cancer. These issues can be understood better if divided under the following sub headings:

- Conventional methods of screening
- Obstacles to widespread screening in low resource settings
- Innovative approaches and lessons learned: progress and pitfalls
- Impact of the vaccines in the developing world : an unprecedented opportunity
- Introductory challenges for the HPV vaccine: public will and political support.

CONVENTIONAL METHODS OF SCREENING

The Pap test is perhaps the best screening test we have developed in medical history. It is easy to administer, minimally invasive, relatively inexpensive, and it detects over 90 percent of precancerous and cancerous lesions of the cervix. However, for Pap tests to be successful, patients must have access to good-quality health-care services, well-run cytology laboratories, and supervised quality control programs, among many other requirements. In addition, a traditional Pap smear screening can be a cumbersome process, requiring 3 visits when an abnormal result occurs: one for the Pap smear, a second for a colposcopy follow-up and biopsy, and the third for treatment such as cryotherapy (freezing of the abnormal tissue).

As one would guess, only a handful of the affluent and educated elite in developing countries have access to these traditional approaches. About 5 percent of women receive Pap smears in developing countries (Katz et al. 2006) as compared to 50–75 percent in developed countries. Such approaches, where only the privileged have access and the people who are at greater risk (such as the underserved and the underprivileged) do not, make a negligible impact on the number of cases and deaths due to cervical cancer in a nation. Fortunately, public officials, health-care professionals, and hospitals are trying to change that and bring about more pragmatic approaches.

OBSTACLES TO WIDESPREAD SCREENING IN LOW-COST SETTINGS

Competing Health-Care Needs

Most developing nations are battling diseases like diarrhea, malaria, tuberculosis, and HIV, which consume most, if not all, of their health-care budget. For example, sub-Saharan Africa holds just over 10 percent of the world's population but 60 percent of the world's population living with HIV. Statistics of catastrophic proportions such as these make it difficult to allocate funds for elective programs like cervical screening, which seem less important in the shadow of the AIDS crisis.

War and Famine

In war-torn developing nations, the victims of famine have lives filled with uncertainties and interruptions to adequate health-care services. When there are acutely inadequate resources to take care of emergencies, routine screenings for healthy people tend to take a back seat. For example, setting up even a rudimentary screening facility for the female population of Darfur, where daily atrocities put their very lives in grave danger, would be a completely improbable proposition.

Poor Health-Care Services

Many health-care centers in developing countries are ill-equipped and have poorly trained and inadequate staff. For example, in Malawi, a country in southeastern Africa, 47 in 100,000 women have cervical cancer, compared to only 8 per 100,000 in the United States. However, in the entire Malawi population of about 13 million people, there is only one pathologist and very few or no facilities to treat cervical cancer.

Poverty and Illiteracy

Knowledge is power. Unfortunately, many women in developing nations, particularly those living in the rural areas, are poorly educated and have no awareness of health issues. In addition, financial constraints create roadblocks to public health education programs and services, meaning that few or no chances exist for these women to gain any knowledge about cervical cancer.

Cultural Barriers

Cultural factors play a pivotal role in health behaviors, attitudes toward illness, and faith in modern medicine versus alternative forms of healing (Freeman 1989, 2003). In many of the developing countries, men, as the main breadwinners, make all of the decisions for their families, including decisions regarding the health care of women. Because females in developing countries are often seen as inferior, their male providers do not take their health-care needs seriously. In addition, cultural barriers cause some women to take shame in pelvic exams, leading to decreased screening and an increase in the number of cases of cervical cancer going undetected.

Professionals' Attitudes Affecting Treatment of Women

In many nations of the world, including the United States, research has been done to document the disparity in quality of care when doctors treat women complaining of the same symptoms as men. Doctors treat men more comprehensively and aggressively, whereas they tend to be more dismissive when treating women. Compounded with the male-dominated societies in some developing countries, women are far less likely to be screened or diagnosed until it is too obvious or, unfortunately, too late for those inflicted with the disease to be treated.

INNOVATIVE APPROACHES AND LESSONS LEARNED: PROGRESS AND PITFALLS

Successful control of cervical cancer rates lies in a country's ability to implement a strong widespread public education and screening program. More established screening protocols and follow-up and treatment programs correlate directly with lower rates of cervical cancer. However, in resource-restricted areas of the world, where there is a lack of an organized population-based cervical cancer screening program, the traditional approaches of the West have failed. These programs have been found to be very laborious and to require significant collaboration to run successfully. It is said that necessity is the mother of invention, and in this case, innovative approaches and alternate methods of screening in developing countries have been initiated with varying degrees of success. The following programs have been attempted by various countries to curb the rising rates of cervical cancer. These provide interesting case studies and shed light on the social, cultural, and economic climate in which the vaccines will be introduced:

Mexico

In Mexico, a nationwide Pap test screening initiative was introduced in the mid 1980s. Even though the program reduced mortality rates from cervical cancer, the results were not as encouraging as one would hope. The reason was a flaw in the system—young women in urban areas were screened repeatedly, whereas older women in their forties (the age when cervical cancer typically develops) had no access to testing. In addition, inadequately trained professionals were using colposcopy—a tool usually reserved for follow-up of abnormal Pap tests—as a diagnostic tool. This led to inaccurate results.

Therefore, the lessons learned here were that screening programs should focus on not only reaching the young women, but more importantly, the at-risk population between the ages of 30 and 50 years, the time period during which precancerous and cancerous lesions peak. Statistics have shown that had this been the case, health officials could have reduced the lifetime risk of cancer in this age group by approximately 25 to 36 percent. Therefore, it is also important to educate and provide adequate training to health-care professionals to perform the necessary tests.

Chile

A widespread Pap testing and education program was developed in Chile in the 1970s. In a recent study, it was shown that more than 80 percent of the married women in Chile have been screened at least once. Since then, the 1990s have seen a marked decline in the mortality rates from cervical cancer in Chile.

Sub-Saharan Africa

South Africa has had its share of trials and tribulations with cervical screening programs; it is one of the regions most affected by cervical cancer in the world. One program in Soweto (a small township in South Africa) is worth mentioning (Leiman 1987). Project Screen Soweto was launched in a major hospital in Soweto by the government and health-care officials to control the increasing incidence of cervical cancer in the region. Cytology-based screening programs were put in place, and laboratory facilities expanded to screen 90,000 Pap smears in one year (Sankaranarayanan et al. 2001). However, lack of a planned population education and fear of burdening the health-care system too rapidly by aggressive campaigning resulted in poor participation by the target population in the program. Hence, no consumer demand was generated. Women remained ignorant of the dangers of cervical cancer, and very few showed up in primary health-care centers for screening. Had the program been run to the fullest extent, it was estimated that it would have detected 6,000 preinvasive and invasive cancers during the five years of this pilot program. The Soweto project reinforces the importance of public education for the success of any widespread screening program. The moral of this story is to educate before implementing any program.

Thailand

Cervical cancer is the most common cancer in women living in Thailand. About 6,000 new cases of cervical cancer are diagnosed in Thailand each year, mainly in women ages 30 to 60. In order to reduce the number of cases (morbidity) and deaths (mortality) from cervical cancer, particularly in rural Thailand, the Thai Ministry of Public Health, in collaboration with a team from the United States, launched a massive campaign to increase public awareness. Around 6,000 women from the Roi-et-Province in Thailand were tested over seven months in village health centers or in district hospitals with a method called visual inspection of the cervix with acetic acid (VIA). Here, acetic acid (vinegar) was applied to the cervix; potentially abnormal areas of the cervix would turn white. The goal was to then treat the abnormal areas with cryotherapy (destruction of tissue by freezing), at the same visit. This was called the one stop "screen and treat approach." Here the investigators were assessing the benefits of a single visit approach as opposed to several visits for screening and treatment

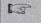 **Widespread public education is key to the success of any preventive program.**

of abnormal Pap smears. Mobile units were dispatched to target women 25–60 years of age. Both VIA testing of the cervix and cryotherapy were highly acceptable to the women. The results of the tests showed that 94 percent of women who had initial abnormal results tested negative for cervical lesions using VIA at one-year follow-up. Such innovative approaches are also being employed in other less-developed areas of the world where government and health officials are grappling with issues of how best to initiate cervical cancer prevention programs. Though not as accurate as routine Pap smears or HPV DNA testing, naked-eye visual inspection of the cervix with acetic-acid wash (VIA) is a good alternative in screening for cervical cancer in poorly resourced locations where Pap testing is just not feasible or practical.

Southeast and East Asia

In Singapore, patients are screened whenever the opportunity arises. This had led to a substantial decrease in cervical cancer cases among the Singapore Indian community, but it has not had the same impact in the Chinese or Malay communities for reasons not quite clear. Singapore has since tried to restructure its screening programs to bring down the disease burden throughout the country. As in Thailand, pilot programs comparing the accuracy of various visual inspection methods are also being tried in Vietnam and Laos. Programs in China are studying the accuracy of Pap smears versus other forms of screening approaches.

India—a Personal Case Study

Having smelled cervical cancer from a distance in the wards of public hospitals in India during my medical school years (advanced cases have a distinct odor due to the presence of dead tissue), this disease hits very close to home. During my visit to Chennai, India, in the summer of 2007,

I decided to explore and learn more about methods that were being tried in rural India to detect cervical cancer. The project that I studied is being funded by the Bill and Melinda Gates Foundation and the International Council on Medical Research at Lyon, France. I met with the doctors at the Adyar Cancer Institute in Chennai who were working on ways to find a simple, culturally acceptable, cost-effective, and reasonably accurate method of cervical screening for rural India. A fascinating pilot program has been in progress since 2000 in three districts, one of which is in the Madurai-Dindigul area of Tamil Nadu in southern India.

Program Background

The same principle of VIA (using acetic acid or vinegar) or VILI (using Lugol's iodine instead of vinegar) and cryotherapy (freezing), as applied in the rural districts of Thailand, were tested here. Around 80,000 women from 113 villages were recruited to participate in the program. One-half was randomly selected to be screened, while the other half was used as controls (the group that was not screened).

Preliminary results have shown that there has been a 30 percent reduction in the incidence and a 42 percent reduction in death from cervical cancer in the group that was screened and treated when compared to the control group (Sankaranarayanan et al. 2004).

One of the most interesting parts of the survey was the patients' responses when they were recruited to participate in the program. The majority of them were agreeable to the screening, but there were a few cynics amidst them. These comments shed some light about the cultural differences and challenges that the vaccines may have to face when they are introduced into the developing world.

- "My husband will leave me for another woman if he finds out that I have cancer, so leave me alone."
- "It is shameful to expose that area when I am feeling fine."
- "My husband says that all the governmental programs are to control fertility."
- "If I have cancer, it is my fault because I must have sinned in my previous birth."
- "If my husband can give me cervical cancer, why don't you talk to him too for screening?" (Good question, I thought.)
- "If I die of cancer that is my fate. Right now, there is no one to take care of my children at home for me to go get this test done."
- If my family finds out that I have cancer, then I won't be allowed to feed my children with my own hands."
- "We are illiterates. You are the doctor. If you say it is good for us, then we will get the test done."
- "My sister died at 40 years of age. We have lost many women in our village to this God's curse. I will get the test done if it will save my life."

India accounts for 20 percent of the world's cases of cervical cancers. Ironically, only a few million Pap tests are done annually in this country where the total population is over one billion. Most of the Pap smears are done in more affluent, private settings. If India could implement a widespread public health cervical screening program to effectively bring down the rates of cervical cancer, it would reduce the global impact of the disease considerably.

THE VACCINES ON THE GLOBAL FRONT: A UNIQUE OPPORTUNITY

Clinical studies have shown that the HPV vaccines can eradicate 70 to 80 percent of the cervical cancer burden on this planet—an impressive feat. Such a claim brings an unprecedented amount of optimism, particularly in the developing nations where the disease burden is the highest, the population most difficult to reach, and the health-care system the weakest. When such a vaccine is introduced into the market, it brings with it the hope to benefit from the vaccine, and at the same time, the challenges and cost to access this "wonder" drug.

Although the eventual release of the HPV vaccine outside of the United States will be met with support if introduced in a culturally sensitive manner, the question remains whether malnutrition and a low-protein diet among the poor in the developing world will stimulate an adequate antibody response. It is also not known if the same vaccine successful in treating American strains of the virus will be effective outside the country as well. Even though HPV type 16 still remains the dominant culprit throughout this world, accounting for over half the cancer-causing strains, followed by HPV type 18 that accounts for another 15–25 percent, regional variations exist (Munoz 2004). Therefore, the impact of the vaccines will also vary across the different regions of the world. So far, multinational studies conducted by both Merck and GSK in more than 33 countries have shown that the current vaccines, *Gardasil*

> ☞ A vaccine could reduce the incidence of cervical cancer by 51 percent if all adolescent girls were vaccinated before their sexual debut.

and *Cervarix*, can be beneficial worldwide as they both are nearly 100 percent effective in covering HPV types 16 and 18. Another study also showed that the vaccine could reduce the incidence of cervical cancer by 51 percent over several years, if all adolescent girls were vaccinated before their sexual debut. The benefits, however, will not be realized for decades—until these girls reach 35 to 50 years of age (Goldie et al. 2004).

The biggest impediment to procuring the vaccines for developing countries, however, is their price. At $120 per dose for a vaccine that requires a set of three doses, the cost is absolutely prohibitive for all but a very few affluent people in developing nations. Even most Americans cannot afford the $360 for the vaccine itself (plus administrative fees) if it is not covered by their health insurance, let alone impoverished people in third-world countries. In order for the vaccine to be affordable to citizens of developing countries, the cost would have to be closer to $1 or $2 per dose as is the case with the hepatitis B vaccine; this has been procured for less than $1 for developing countries. The GAVI Alliance (Global Alliance for Vaccines and Immunizations)—a partnership among national governments, the Bill and Melinda Gates Foundation, the World Bank, the vaccine industry, public health institutions, and nongovernmental organizations—provides financial and technical assistance to countries where the gross national income is less than $1,000 per capita. GAVI is in the process of reviewing the HPV vaccine to see if it should be added to the list of vaccines that have already been approved by it.

There is a compelling need for prevention of cervical cancer in the developing world. It is estimated by the International Agency for Research on Cancer that, if nothing is done to raise the rates of screening and treatment and lower the viral spread in the developing world between now and 2050, the incidence of death due to cervical cancer will reach 1 million people per year—four times the current fatality rate. This anticipated rise is attributed to the increase in population, increased sexual activity, and industrialization of rural areas. Industrialization will lead to higher rates of cigarette smoking, decreased physical activity, and increased consumption of more refined and less homegrown foods, all of which lead to a more sedentary and unhealthy lifestyle—a risk factor for cervical cancer in the presence of HPV infections. However, the general consensus among doctors and other health-care professionals in the international community is that the vaccine has a very narrow spectrum of coverage, and if more cancer-causing strains were included, a larger portion of the world's population could be served better. All the health officials to whom I spoke were also hopeful that the vaccine studies in males, soon to be released, would prove that the vaccine is beneficial in boys and men so that they could also be vaccinated. They unanimously felt that vaccinating boys would reduce the HPV pool in circulation and not put all the focus on girls alone. In addition, it would send the message to men that they have to take responsibility in preventing this disease even though it does not affect them as much as it does their female partners. Ultimately, the best approach might be to vaccinate

> ☞ The best approach to reduce cervical cancer rates in developing countries would be to vaccinate all preadolescent girls (and, ideally, boys) and screen women at least once between the ages of 30 and 50 as a starting point.

all preadolescent girls (and, ideally, boys) and continue to screen women at least once between the ages of 30 and 50. A first screening at 30–50 years of age is a reasonable target for cervical cancer control programs in countries with limited resources (PATH 2000). In addition, the health officials were quick to point out that the vaccine would be most beneficial if it were not just preventive but also helped in treating existing HPV infections. Streamlining the series to one dose as opposed to three would also ensure higher participation and success rates. Such possibilities are currently under study.

INTRODUCTORY CHALLENGES FOR THE HPV VACCINES: POLITICAL WILL AND PUBLIC SUPPORT

The HPV vaccines bring with it an arena of sociopolitically charged debates on sexual health, sexuality, and sexually transmitted infections. The much-anticipated arrival of the vaccine has finally come to fruition, and now the next challenge lies in ensuring its universal access and getting it to the parts of the world where it is needed most.

Fortunately, the work of procuring the vaccine for the developing world is well on its way. Advocates from immunization, cancer, and reproductive health sectors—organizations that do not traditionally work together—are now discussing the possibility of combining their resources to ensure that the vaccine is made available to developing countries as soon as possible. In December 2006, the World Health Organization released a set of guidelines to help health workers around the world prepare for the vaccine's introduction. The exact date of release is yet to be determined.

One would think that if the vaccine tipped off such a whirlwind of ethical debate in the United States, it must be even more culturally challenging to introduce it in countries such as India, where the mind set is more conservative and people are not as health conscious. Surprisingly, people there, particularly in villages, seem to be more accepting of the vaccine's adoption than Americans. One physician working in a rural area of India said, "People here are illiterates. The visual images of death of a friend or a relative and the destruction of families that they have witnessed from this deadly disease trump all other considerations and have them convinced enough to get the vaccine. They are not worried about issues of the vaccine being administered to young girls before their sexual debut as much as they are concerned about how long will it be before the vaccine is available, and will it be affordable?"

Ensuring universal access to cervical cancer prevention, screening, and treatment services will be the key to reducing cervical cancer worldwide. If due attention is not given to reaching the poorer women in the world, the new vaccine will fail to bridge the gap of health inequities and realize the goals of reducing cervical cancer worldwide. With some creativity, flexibility, and well-focused use of resources, the fight against cervical cancer can be won. Some of the challenges that the global community could face during the worldwide introduction of the vaccine include the following:

Vaccine Supply

Without knowing the demand, it will be hard to predict if adequate amounts of vaccines will be available to meet it. Pharmaceutical companies are unlikely to invest in expanding their manufacturing capabilities and moving toward a cost structure that would produce low profit margins. Phased introduction of the vaccine in small test areas would be more practical than nationwide start-ups and would greatly help forecast demand. It would also provide models to refine the system to local settings.

Delivery Methods for the Vaccines

Setting up mobile outreach services is important as distance, cost of transport, and lost time are significant deterrents to any health prevention program. One stop screen-and-treat or single-visit programs are key components to cervical cancer prevention. It is also important to select women from the appropriate target population of 30–50 years, the age group in which cervical cancer is more prevalent.

In countries such as the United States, school-based immunization programs work effectively because enrollment is high. However, in developing countries, where only a small number of girls attend school at nine years (the youngest age when the vaccine can be given and by which time many girls have already dropped out of school in these countries), access to this age population becomes difficult. In such cases, alternate programs such as national immunization campaigns must be designed to cater to the targeted population.

Public Education

One of the most important, basic considerations in public education would be how to present this new vaccine. Social, cultural, and religious contexts will have to be considered. Providing a vaccine to preadolescent girls against cancer that may occur decades down the road poses several challenges. Vaccine promotion and incentive programs should be packaged with other adolescent health services. They should address the needs of this age group, because in many cultures, young girls cannot easily visit a reproductive health clinic without raising questions about their character and morality. All the benefits and limitations of the vaccines must be explained with emphasis on the fact that screening programs will still remain a necessary component of the program because the vaccine is not proven to be 100 percent effective against all types of cancer-causing strains.

Monitoring and evaluating the impact of the vaccine will also be essential, as the full benefits of the vaccine will only be realized much further down the road. This is critical, as many people may expect immediate results and get discouraged if they do not see a reduction in the total number of incidence and deaths in their communities within a few years.

In addition, the primary goal of any global policy should be to not only improve cancer screening but also to restrict the spread of HPV. In this context, it is important to acknowledge the role that sex plays in the spread of HPV and cervical cancer, even if the topic is taboo in many developing countries. Even though sex outside of marriage is not tolerated in many countries, the rate of premarital and extramarital sex remains high in those countries. In cultures where men have more sexual freedom than women, it becomes all the more important to educate both men and women about the spread and natural history of the virus. For example, Uganda embarked on a campaign known as ABC (abstinence, being faithful, and condom use) to help prevent the spread of HIV. A similar campaign can also be tried for HPV education. A campaign to provide information about the HPV vaccine and cervical screening programs should be promoted prominently in addition to campaigns promoting safe sexual behavior such as condom use and abstinence. In areas where illiteracy is high, awareness can be increased through culturally sensitive programs such as stage dramas and puppet shows. Such measures have been employed to curtail HIV/AIDS in high-risk areas, so there is no reason why similar measures cannot work for HPV. A strong partnership between the community leaders and local health services will also help educate and provide valuable material and social support to the community. Likewise, in order to ensure that the necessary priority is given to the vaccine on the global public agenda, health officials and policy-makers should also be educated with the facts about the human papillomavirus and vaccine, including lessons learned from prior vaccine introduction initiatives.

Financing

Financing is going to be the deciding factor in how long the lag time will be for introducing the vaccine in the developing world. Mobilization of both international and national organizations in the public and private sector will be crucial to obtaining global financial support for HPV prevention programs and vaccines. Currently, *Gardasil* and *Cervarix* are the only HPV vaccines on the market, but other drug manufacturers are developing their own vaccines to create competition and keep the prices down. It is necessary to act quickly to finance this effort, as even a delay of five years in procuring the vaccine for the global community would cost another 1.5–2 million deaths from cervical cancer. A good start along this line is Merck's intent to donate 3 million doses of the vaccine to the lowest income nations in the near future. GSK has also submitted a file on its cervical cancer vaccine *Cervarix* to the World Health Organization for prequalification, which in turn could speed the delivery of the new vaccine to developing countries as early as possible. This is an effort to eliminate the historical 15–20-year delay for the new vaccine to become available in countries where it is needed the most. GSK will provide its cervical cancer vaccine at preferential prices to low-income countries. Although such philanthropic moves are very admirable, measures have to be taken to ensure that plans are in place for sustained delivery of the vaccines. If not, it will raise expectations and be a potential cause for resentment in the international community.

Advocacy

Advocacy will be important to influence policy-making, inform public opinion, correct misperceptions, and mobilize resources. Strong international public health advocacy at the highest level led to the procurement of the Hepatitis B vaccine at highly discounted rates for the developing world. (It is about 75 cents per vaccine dose in India.)

Cervical cancer in the developing world is a reflection of the global inequity of socioeconomic conditions. Too many women live in poverty and have died of invasive cervical cancer. In 1991, Dr. Samuel Broder, then the Director of the U.S. National Cancer Institute said, "Poverty is a carcinogen." If due attention is not given to reaching poorer women, the new vaccine will contribute to the increase in health inequities, rather than contributing to the goal of universal access to preventive care against cervical cancer. For the first time, we have the availability of an effective and safe vaccine that offers hope for reducing the global burden of cervical cancer. Although achieving broad coverage of young adolescents, negotiating pricing, and securing financing will be a challenge, the vaccine's potential to save millions of lives offers solace. An integrated approach that includes screening and vaccination will, most likely, prevent the greatest number of deaths due to cervical cancer. Let us hope that the introduction of the HPV vaccine will help fulfill its goal of making each and every woman be "one less" in the statistics for cervical cancer.

KEY FACTS

- Cervical cancer affects an estimated 500,000 women worldwide each year and is responsible for more that 250,000 deaths.
- If current trends continue, there will be more than 1 million new cases by the year 2050.
- Simple, inexpensive, and cost-effective screening programs can detect precancerous lesions in nearly 90 percent of cases. Cervical cancer can be prevented if these lesions are treated early in the disease process.

- Cooperation and collaboration between several governmental and nongovernmental agencies are required to introduce the vaccine into the developing world.

- Vaccinating all preadolescents and screening women at least once between the ages of 30 and 50 will significantly reduce the mortality rates from cervical cancer.

- Every woman should be entitled to cervical screening at least once in her lifetime.

PRATHIBHA'S STORY

I would like to leave you with a stirring story of one woman's experience in India that goes to show how prevention efforts can save lives.

This is a story that has been adapted from *Women's Stories, Women's Lives: Experiences with Cervical Cancer Screening and Treatment,* a publication of the Alliance for Cervical Cancer Prevention and based on the work of the International Agency for Research on Cancer.

Prathibha, a 37-year-old woman, lives in Maharashtra State, India. Talk among women at her local water well, (India's equivalent of our office coffee machine), alerted her to the fact that there was a team conducting cervical cancer screening in her area. Although Prathibha would have liked to linger at the well to chat with the other women, she had to hurry back home because her mother-in-law was waiting for her. When Prathibha arrived at her house, she was shocked to see two women from a cancer hospital talking to her husband. After he gave them permission, they interviewed her, got her history, and told her about cervical cancer. They informed her that it was common in women in her region, but if it was detected early, it was a preventable disease. She was still not sure about getting screened, and she knew she would have to get her husband and mother-in-law to approve her going to the ad-hoc clinic set up in the village. But the village elder, the *panchayat,* whose mother had died of cervical cancer when he was 10 years old, had already given his tacit approval, so her husband and mother-in-law agreed. The test was free, and after the health workers explained the procedure, they recommended that Prathibha undergo the test even if she had no symptoms.

Prathibha's test results were positive for severely abnormal cells. She was dumbfounded—she had felt no symptoms and was perfectly healthy. She was hesitant to undergo the recommended Loop Electrosurgical Excision Procedure (LEEP) at the cancer hospital, but after doing so, she found out that the LEEP was positive for cancer, and the doctor advised she get a hysterectomy. Prathibha was now in total shock. She could not believe that she was in such a dire predicament—going from feeling perfectly healthy to being diagnosed with cancer in a matter of days. However, after being consoled by a friend, she underwent the hysterectomy.

While in the hospital, Prathibha talked to another woman who had advanced cancer. The woman was very upset and worried about what would happen to her children if she died. Prathibha thought, "Listening to her, I thought how lucky I was to get the opportunity to attend the program. These people saved my life. They have not only saved a woman but they have saved the mother of a small child. If I did not attend the clinic, what would have happened to me? This thought frightens me even now. I am lucky that I live in the village of Osmanabad District, which has been selected for this program. I am thankful to these people, who put in so much effort to convince me to get tested and prevent cancer. They saved my life and my family."

This story clearly illustrates the complexity of women's lives, and the many obstacles—husband, mother-in-law, and village elders—to be overcome before instituting a widespread screening program. It also shows the challenges posed by long journeys to the nearest clinic, local myths and fears, and poor health services that prevent women from being screened for cervical cancer.

In the Western world, a diagnosis of cervical cancer no doubt brings with it feelings of fear and horror, but a fear and horror that is tempered with hope and survival. Unfortunately, in the developing world, this is not the case. Many women continue to die from the ravages of cervical cancer. We can only wish that the introduction of the HPV vaccines will help to raise public awareness, and that millions of women will learn to battle a disease that, for the present, they do not even know they can control.

GLOSSARY

Ablative procedure: A technique used to remove tissue through radio wave frequency.

Acetowhitening: The process by which HPV infected cells turn white when they are painted with acetic acid (vinegar).

Adenocarcinoma: Cancer that arises from the glandular epithelium. An example is cervical adenocarcinoma.

Adjuvant: A pharmacological substance that is added to a drug to enhance its effect.

AIDS: Acquired immune deficiency syndrome. A disease caused by the HIV virus in which the body's immune system breaks down.

Anal: Pertaining to the anus.

Anal cancer: Cancer of the epithelial layer of the anal canal.

Anogenital: Pertaining to the anus and the external genitals.

Anoscopy: A procedure in which a scope is used to examine the inside of the anus.

Antigenic: A substance that stimulates the production of antibodies.

Anus: The terminal opening of the digestive tract.

ASCUS: Atypical squamous cells of undetermined significance. A mildly abnormal Pap smear that may or may not be of any clinical significance.

Atypical: Not conforming to any specific type or strain.

Autoinoculation: An infection from an organism such as a virus that spreads from one part of the body to another.

Basal cells: The cells in the lower-most layer of the epithelium.

Benign: A condition that does not lead to cancer and has a favorable outcome.

Bethesda system: A system used to classify abnormal Pap smears.

Biopsy: The procedure of removing a piece of tissue for the diagnosis and treatment.

Cancer: Uncontrolled growth of abnormal cells.

Capsid: The protein envelope of a virus.

Carcinogen: A cancer-causing substance.

Carcinoma: A cancerous tumor.

Carcinoma in situ: A precancerous condition that may progress to invasive cancer if not treated in time.

Cervarix: An HPV vaccine, manufactured by GlaxoSmithKline, that offers protection against HPV types 16 and 18.

Cervical: Pertaining to the cervix.

Cervical intraepithelial neoplasias (CIN): A condition in which abnormal cells of the cervix may progress to cancer if left untreated. Also known as dysplasia. The CIN system is one of the methods to classify abnormal Pap smears.

Cervix: The opening of the uterus.

Chemotherapy: A treatment where a chemical or chemicals bind to tumor cells and kill them.

Chlamydia: A type of bacteria that is sexually transmitted.

Circumcision: A surgical procedure that removes the loose skin (foreskin) that covers the "head" (glans) of the penis.

Clinical trial: A series of unproven treatments used to evaluate the effectiveness and safety of a drug or vaccine using informed human subjects.

Cofactor: Something (for example a substance or a bacteria) that aids another factor (such as the HPV virus) in causing disease.

Cohort: A generational group of people as defined in statistics or demographics.

Colposcope: A lighted, magnifying instrument that is usually used to magnify and view the cervix.

Colposcopy: A procedure where a colposcope is used to directly examine the cervix and vagina under magnification.

Columnar cells: Tall cells that line organs and produce mucous.

Condom: A thin sheath usually made of latex or polyurethane that is placed over an erect penis just before intercourse.

Condyloma acuminata: Genital warts.

Conization: A procedure in which a scalpel or a laser is used to remove a cone-shaped piece of the cervix containing the area with abnormal cells for diagnosis and treatment purposes.

Conjunctiva: A thin transparent tissue that covers the lining of the inner eyelids and the white part of the eyeballs.

Control group: A group in an experiment or a clinical trial that does not receive a new treatment or a procedure and is compared with the group that receives the new treatment or the procedure in order to validate the results of the test.

Cross-infection: The transmission of infectious disease between patients and staff because of a poor barrier.

Cross-protection: A decreased risk of infection from one or more strains that are not targeted by the vaccines.

Cryotherapy/cryosurgery: A method of super-freezing and killing cancerous and precancerous cells.

Cutaneous: Pertaining to skin.

Dental dam: A rectangular sheet usually made of latex that is used as a barrier method during oral and anal sex.

DNA: Deoxyribonucleic acid. It carries an organism's genetic information and is capable of replication.

Dysplasia: A condition in which abnormal cells may progress to cancer if left untreated.

Ectocervix: The portion of the cervix that is exposed to the vagina and is lined by squamous cells.

Endocervical curettage: A procedure in which scrapings from the endocervical canal are obtained with the help of a curette (spoon-shaped instrument) and then tested for the presence of abnormal cells.

Endocervix: The mucous membrane lining the canal of the cervix.

Epidemiology: The branch of medicine that studies the causes, distribution, and control of diseases among various populations.

Epithelium: The layer of cells that lines several organs.

External radiation therapy: Radiation therapy that uses a machine located outside of the body to deliver high-energy beam at cancer cells.

Gardasil: An HPV vaccine, manufactured by Merck, that protects against HPV types 6, 11, 16, and 18. It has been approved for use in the United States for girls as young as 9 years of age.

Herpes: A viral disease that can affect skin or mucous membranes

HIV: Human immunodeficiency virus that causes AIDS.

HSIL: High-grade squamous intraepithelial lesions. A diagnosis of moderately to severely abnormal cells on a Pap smear.

Hybrid capture II: The commercially available test that detects high risk HPVs.

Hysterectomy: A major surgery that involves removal of the cervix and the uterus.

Incidence rate: The number of new cases during the specified period of time.

In situ: In the original place or arrangement. For example, when the abnormal cells have not broken through the basement membrane and are in their original place.

Interferon: A naturally occurring substance that stimulates the immune system.

Internal radiation therapy: A type of cancer therapy in which sealed radioactive material is placed directly in or close to a cancerous site.

Intraepithelial: Within the layer of cells that forms the skin layer or the lining of an organ.

Intraepithelial neoplasias: A condition where intraepithelial cells become abnormal, most often as a result of HPV infection.

Invasive cancer: A condition in which cancer cells have invaded the basement membrane and spread to the underlying tissue.

Keratin: A tough and insoluble protein that forms a major component of structures like skin and hair.

Keratinization: The process of formation of a hard coating on epithelial cells due to production of keratin.

Labia majora: The two prominent outer folds of skin that are present on either side of the opening of the vagina.

Labia minora: The two inner lips of skin folds that encircle the clitoris and opening of the vagina.

Larynx: The voice box.

Laser surgery: A procedure in which a narrow beam of high-energy light is used to destroy abnormal cells.

LEEP: Loop electrosurgical excision procedure. An electrical current is passed through a wire loop that is used to remove a very precise amount of abnormal tissue from the cervix.

Lesion: Abnormal change in a tissue usually due to a disease process.

LSIL: Low-grade squamous intraepithelial lesions. This means that mildly abnormal cells are found on the Pap smear.

Metastasis: Spread of cancer from the original site to another part of the body.

Mucosal: Relating to mucous membrane, such as in the vagina or mouth.

Neoplasia: Means new growth in Greek. It is the abnormal growth of cells resulting in a tumor or cancer.

Oncogenic: Tending to cause the development of cancer.

Opt out: To exempt oneself from participating in particular program.

Oral: Of the mouth.

Papilloma: A benign tumor that resembles a finger-like projection, usually associated with HPV.

Pap smear: Smear obtained from the cervix, anus, or vagina.

Pap test: The observation or examination of cells obtained during a Pap smear.

Penile cancer: Cancer of the penis.

Perianal: Area surrounding the anus.

Precursor: That which heralds or precedes.

Prepuce: The fold of skin that acts like a hood over the male penis or the female clitoris.

Prevalence rate: The number of people in a population that have an illness or a disease at any given point of time.

Prognosis: A prediction of whether a disease will improve or worsen.

Radiation therapy: The medical use of radiation to treat cancer.

Recurrent: Return of a condition after treatment.

Recurrent respiratory papillomatosis: The recurrent growth of benign tumors in the airway tract.

Risk factor: A condition that increases a person's chance of getting an illness or a disease.

Sensitivity: The sensitivity of a test is its ability to detect people with a disease.

Squamous: From Latin squama, meaning "scale." Flat cells of the skin or epithelium.

Squamous cell carcinoma: Cancer of the squamous cells of the skin or epithelium.

Staging: A coded format that is used to determine the severity of the cancer.

Stridor: A high-pitched breathing sound caused by partial blockage of air passages.

Subclinical: An illness or infection that stays below the surface and does not have any clinical manifestations.

Therapeutic: Treatment that has healing powers.

Titer: Measurement of the concentration of a substance.

Topical: Pertaining to a particular surface area.

Trachelectomy: From Greek trachel, menaing "neck." It refers to surgical removal of the neck of the uterus, which is the cervix. It is also known as cervicectomy.

Transformation zone: The junction where squamous cells and columnar cells meet.

Transmission: The act of passing on an infection from one person to another.

Urethra: The tube that connects the urinary bladder to the outside and discharges urine and (in males) semen.

Uterus: The major female reproductive organ, where a developing baby is carried prior to birth. Also known as the womb.

Vaccine: A preparation that is used to build immunity against a particular disease.

Vagina: The birth canal.

VAIN: Vaginal intraepithelial neoplasia. The presence of abnormal vaginal squamous cells, which could progress to cancer if not treated in time.

VIN: Vulvar intraepithelial neoplasias. The presence of abnormal vulvar squamous cells, which could progress to cancer if not treated in time.

Virus: From Latin virus meaning "poison." It is an infectious agent that thrives only in a living cell.

Vulva: The region of the external genital organs of the female.

Vulvar cancer: Cancer of the vulva.

Warts: Benign cauliflower-like growths caused as a result of HPV infections.

Internet Resources

One can never be careful enough about the source of material when it comes to health-related questions. The Internet can be like a double-edged sword; while being a great resource for medical information, it can also be a haven for misinformation that can cause needless worries. Therefore, one has to choose resources very carefully. In order to aid you in this endeavor, I have included a list of Web sites that I believe you will find to be reliable and to provide user-friendly information. They are as follows:

About.com:
http://www.womenshealth.about.com

A.D.A.M. Medical Encyclopedia:
http://www.nlm.nih.gov/medlineplus/encyclopedia.html

American Cancer Society:
http://www.cancer.org

American College of Obstetricians and Gynecologists:
http://www.acog.org

American Social Health Association—National HPV and Cervical Cancer Prevention Resource Center:
http://www.ashastd.org **or for teens,** *http://www.iwannaknow.org*

Centers for Disease Control:
http://www.cdc.gov/std/hpv/STDFact-HPV-vaccine.htm

FDA Office of Women's Health:
http://www.fda.gov/womens/getthefacts/hpv.html

National Cancer Institute:
http://www.cancer.gov

National Cervical Cancer Coalition:
http://www.nccc-online.org

National Institutes of Health:
http://www.nih.gov

National Women's Health Information Center:
http://www.4women.gov

Planned Parenthood:
http://www.plannedparenthood.org

OTHER USEFUL WEB SITES

National Immunization Program:
Email: *nipinfo@cdc.gov*
Web site: *http://www.cdc.gov/nip/*
Provides information about vaccines, including precautions and contraindications for immunization and vaccine shortages.

Recurrent Respiratory Papillomatosis Foundation:
http://www.rrpf.org

Medical Dictionaries:
Medical and Biological (World Health Organization)
http://www.who.int/hlt/virtuallibrary/English/diction.htm#Medical

Online Support Groups:
http://www.ashastd.org/hpv/hpv_community.cfm

Global news on cervical cancer vaccines:
http://www.path.org/projects/cervical_cancer_vaccine.php
Gives basic information and fact sheets as well as some detail on PATH programs introducing HPV vaccine in developing countries.

REFERENCES

AUTHOR'S NOTE

Altman LK. Sex Infections Found in Quarter of Teenage Girls. *New York Times.* March 12, 2008. Available online at http://query.nytimes.com/gst/fullpage .html?res=9507E6D6113BF931A25750C0A96E9C8B63&sec=&spon. Accessed May 2008.

CHAPTER 1: THE HPV VACCINE CONTROVERSY: SCIENCE VERSUS FAITH

American Social Health Association. HPV Vaccine Access in the US. Available online at http://www.ashastd.org/pdfs/hpv_faq_032007.pdf. Accessed March 2008.

Association of Immunization Managers, Position Statement: School and Child Care Immunization Requirements. Available online at http://www .immunizationmanagers.org/pdfs/SchoolrequirementsFINAL.pdf. Accessed March 2008.

Bernard EJ. An HPV Vaccine—What It Might Really Mean. *aidsmap news.* October 24, 2005. Available online at http://www.aidsmap.com/en/news/ 3429199D-5FE5-4795-B0E6-CD957617C160.asp. Accessed March 2008.

Bleakley A, Hennessy M, Fishbein M. Public Opinion on Sex Education in US Schools. *Arch Pediatr Adolesc Med* 2006;160: 151–1156.

Blum D, Knudson M, Henig RM. *A Field Guide for Science Writers.* 2nd ed. New York: Oxford University Press; 2006

The Centers for Disease Control and Prevention (CDC). *2003 Youth Risk Behavior Survey.* Atlanta (GA): Department of Health and Human Services, Centers for Disease Control and Prevention.

Charo RA. J.D. Politics, Parents, and Prophylaxis—Mandating HPV Vaccination in the United States. *NEJM*2007;357-19:1905–1908.

Colgrove J. *State of Immunity: The Politics of Vaccination in Twentieth Century America.* Berkeley: University of California Press; 2006.

Dailard, C. Legislating Against Arousal: The Growing Divide Between Federal Policy and Teenage Sexual Behavior. *Guttmacher Policy Review* 2006;9(3):12–16.

Elliott, MT. House Committee Hears Testimony over HPV Vaccine. *The Daily Texan* online. http://media.www.dailytexanonline.com. Accessed April 2008.

Gostin LO, DeAngelis CD. Mandatory HPV Vaccination Public Health vs Private Wealth.*JAMA* 2007;297:1921–1923.

Grady D. Second Opinion; A Vital Discussion, Clouded. *The New York Times.* March 6, 2007. http://www.nytimes.com/2007/03/06/health/06seco.html? fta=y. Accessed April 2008.

Myers ER, McCrory DC, Nanda K, Bastian L, Matchar DB. Mathematical Model for the Natural History of Human Papillomavirus Infection and Cervical Carcinogenesis. *Am J Epidemiol* 2000;151:1158–1171.

National Institutes of Health (NIH). Cervical Cancer. NIH Consensus Statement 1996; 14:1–38.

Orenstein WA, Hinman AR. The Immunization System in the United States—the Role of School Immunization laws.*Vaccine* 1999;17:Suppl 3:S19–S24.

Pollitt K. Virginity or Death! *The Nation.* May 30, 2005. http://www.thenation.com /doc/20050530/pollitt. Accessed April 2008.

Rubin R. Merck Drops its Push for Vaccine Mandate. *USA Today.* February 20, 2007. http://www.usatoday.com/news/health/2007-02-20-merck-hpv-vaccine_x.htm. Accessed April 2008.

Rubin R. Vaccines: Mandate or choice? *USA Today.* Feburary 7, 2007. http:// findarticles.com/p/articles/mi_kmusa/is_/ai_n18649822. Accessed April 2008.

Saarman E. How We Got the Controversial HPV Vaccine. Discover. *Health and Medicine.* May 17, 2007. http://discovermagazine.com/topics/health-medicine/infectious-diseases. Accessed April 2008.

Salmon DA, Teret SP, MacIntyre CR, et al. Compulsory Vaccination and Conscientious or Philosophical Exemptions: Past, Present, and Future. *Lancet* 2006;367:436–442.

Saul S, Pollack A. Furor on Rush to Require Cervical Cancer Vaccine. *The New York Times.* February 17, 2007. http://www.nytimes.com/2007/02/17/health/17 vaccine.html. Accessed April 2008.

Should HPV vaccination be mandatory for all adolescents? Editorial *Lancet* 2006; 368:1212.

Temte, JL. HPV Vaccine: A Cornerstone of Female Health. *American Family Physician* 2007;75. http://www.aafp.org/afp/20070101/editorials.html. Accessed April 2008.

Verweij M, Dawson A. Ethical Principles for Collective Immunization Programmes. *Vaccine* 2004;22:3122–3126.

Walboomers JM, Jacobs MV, Manos MM, et al. Human Papillomavirus is a Necessary Cause of Invasive Cervical Cancer Worldwide. *J Pathol* 1999;189:12–19.

Weinstock H, Berman S, Cates W Jr. Sexually Transmitted Diseases among American Youth: Incidence and Prevalence Estimates, 2000. *Perspect Sex Reprod Health* 2004;36:6–10.

Chapter 2: HPV Transmission and Natural History: A "Silent" Epidemic

American Cancer Society (ACS). Frequently Asked Questions About Human Papilloma Virus (HPV) Vaccines. www.cancer.org. Accessed March 2008.

American Social Health Association. Human Papilloma Virus. http://www .ashastd.org/hpv/hpv_learn_fastfacts.cfm. Accessed April 2008.

Bartholomew DA. Human Papilloma Virus Infection in Adolescents: A Rational Approach. *Adolescent Medicine Clinics*2004;15(3):569–595.

Bosch FX, de Sanjosé S. Human Papillomavirus and Cervical Cancer—Burden and Assessment of Causality. *J Natl Cancer Inst Monogr* 2003;31:3–13.

Centers for Disease Control (CDC). Genital HPV Infection—CDC Fact Sheet. http://www.cdc.gov/std/HPV/STDFact-HPV.htm. Accessed April 2008.

Cubie HA, Plumstead M, Zhang W, de Jesus O, Duncan LA, Stanley MA. Presence of Antibodies to Human Papillomavirus Virus-like Particles (VLPs) in 11–13-year-old schoolgirls. *Med Virol* 1998;56(3):210–216.

Duensing S, Munger K. Mechanisms of Genomic Instability in Human Cancer: Insights from Studies with Human Papillomavirus Oncoproteins. *Int J Cancer* 2004;109:157–162.

Frega A, Cenci M, Stentella P, Cipriano L, De Ioris A, Alderisio M, Vecchione A. Human Papillomavirus in Virgins and Behaviour at Risk. *Cancer Letters* 2008;194(1):21–24.

Gravitt PE, Jamshidi R. Diagnosis and Management of Oncogenic Cervical Human Papillomavirus Infection. *Infect Dis Clin North Am* 2005;19: 439–458

Greer CE, Wheeler CM, Ladner MB, et al. Human Papillomavirus (HPV) Type Distribution and Serological Response to HPV Type 6 Virus-like Particles in Patients with Genital Warts. *J Clin Microbiol* 1995;33:2058–2063.

Ho GY, Bierman R, Beardsley L, Chang CJ, Burk RD. Natural History of Cervico-vaginal Papillomavirus Infection in Young Women. *N Engl J Med* 1998; 338:423–428.

Koutsky LA, Kiviat NB. Genital Human Papillomavirus. In: Holmes KK, Sparling PF, Mardh PA, et al, eds. *Sexually Transmitted Diseases*. New York: McGraw-Hill; 1999:347–359.

Krejci EB, Sanchez ML. Genital Human Papillomavirus Infections. *Clinics in Family Practice* 2005;7:1.

Mandell GL, Bennett JE, Dolin R. *Principles and Practice of Infectious Diseases,* 6th ed. Philadelphia: Elsevier Churchill Livingstone; 2005.

Mayoclinic.com. HPV infections. http://mayoclinic.com/. Accessed March 2008.

Moscicki AB, Shiboski S, Broering J, et al. The Natural History of Human Papillomavirus Infection as Measured by Repeated DNA Testing in Adolescent and Young Women. *J Pediatr* 1998;132:277–284.

National Cancer Institute. Human Papillomavirus and Cancer: Questions and answers. http://www.cancer.gov/. Accessed March 2008.

Palefsky J, *What Your Doctor May Not Tell You About, HPV and Abnormal Pap Smears.* New York: Warner Books Inc; 2002.

Peyton CL, Gravitt PE, Hunt WC, et al. Determinants of Genital Human Papillomavirus Detection in a US Population. *J Infect Dis* 2001;183:1554–1564.

Puranen M, Syrjanen K, Syrjanen S. Transmission of Genital Human Papillomavirus Infections Is Unlikely through the Floor and Seats of Humid Dwellings in Countries of High-Level Hygiene. *Scand J Infect Dis* 1996;28 (3):243–246.

Reeves WC, Ruparelia SS, Swanson KI, Derkay CS, Marcus A, Unger ER. National Registry for Juvenile-Onset Recurrent Respiratory Papillomatosis. *Arch Otolaryngol Head Neck Surg* 2003;129:976–982.

Rice PS, Cason J, Best JM, Banatvala JE. High Risk Genital Papillomavirus Infections Are Spread Vertically.*Rev Med Virol* 1999 January-March;9(1): 15–21.

Vermund SH, Bhatta MP. Papillomavirus Infections. In: Cohen J, Powderly WG, eds. *Infectious Diseases*, 2nd ed. New York: Mosby, An Imprint of Elsevier; 2004.

de Villiers EM, Fauquet C, Broker TR, Bernard HU, zur Hausen H. Classification of Papillomaviruses. *Virology* 2004;324:17–27.

Watts DH, Koutsky LA, Holmes KK, et al. Low Risk of Perinatal Transmission of Human Papillomavirus: Results from a Prospective Cohort Study. *Am J Obstet Gynecol* 1998;178:365–373.

Winer RL, Hughes JP, Feng Q, et al. Condom Use and the Risk of Genital Human Papillomavirus Infection in Young Women. *N Engl J Med* 2006;354:2645–2654.

Winer RL, Lee SK, Hughes JP, Adam DE, Kiviat NB, Koutsky LA. Genital Human Papillomavirus Infection: Incidence and Risk Factors in a Cohort of Female University Students. *Am J Epidemiol* 2003 Feb 1;157(3):218–226:

Woodman CBJ, Collins SI, Young LS. The Natural History of Cervical HPV Infection: Unresolved Issues. *Nature Reviews Cancer* 2007;7:11-22

World Health Organization (WHO). IARC Monograph on the Evaluation of Carcinogenic Risks to Humans: Human Papillomaviruses. 1995. Lyons, France: IARC; 2000.

CHAPTER 3: RISK FACTORS AND TESTING: KNOWLEDGE IS POWER

American Academy of Family Physicians. Human Papillomavirus Testing. http:// familydoctor.org/. Accessed April 2008

American Academy of Family Physicians. Summary of Policy Recommendations for Periodic Health Examinations. November 1996, Revision 5.1.http:// familydoctor.org/. Accessed December 2001.

American Cancer Society (ACS). Guidelines for Early Detection of Cancer. http://www.cancer.org/docroot/ped/content/ped_2_3x_acs_cancer_detection_ guidelines_36.asp. Accessed April 2008.

American Cancer Society (ACS). Pap Smear Guidelines. http://www.cancer.org/ docroot/CRI/content/CRI_2_4_2X_can_cervical_cancer_be_prevented_8.asp. Accessed April 2008.

American Cancer Society (ACS). Risk Factors for Cervical Cancer. http://www .cancer.org/docroot/CRI/content/CRI_2_4_2X_What_are_the_risk_factors_for _cervical_cancer_8.asp. Accessed April 2008.

American Social Heath Association. New HPV Tests. http://www.ashastd.org/ hpv/hpv_learn_women.cfm. Accessed April 2008.

Barton SE, Maddox PH, Jenkins D, et al. Effect of Cigarette Smoking on Cervical Epithelial Immunity: A Mechanism for Neoplastic Change? *Lancet* 1988;2:652–4.

Boggs, W. Smoking Multiplies HPV-16-Related Cervical Cancer Risk. *Cancer Epidemiol Biomarkers Prev* 2006;15:2141–2147.

Bosch FX, de Sanjosé S. Human Papillomavirus and Cervical Cancer—Burden and Assessment of Causality. *J Natl Cancer Inst Monogr* 2003;31:3–13.

Cancer Research UK. Cervical Cancer Risks and Causes http://www.cancerhelp .org.uk/. Accessed March 2008.

Castellsagué X, Muñoz N. Cofactors in Human Papillomavirus Carcinogenesis—Role of Parity, Oral Contraceptives, and Tobacco Smoking. *JNCI* 2003;(31), 20–28.

Centers for Disease Control and Prevention (CDC). Tracking the Hidden Epidemic Trends in STDs in the United States. http://www.cdc.gov/std/Trends2000/Trends2000.pdf. Accessed April 2008.

Coker AL, Bond SM, Williams A, Gerasimova T, Pirisi L. Active and Passive Smoking, High-Risk Human Papillomaviruses and Cervical Neoplasia. *Cancer Detection and Prevention* May 2002;26(2):121–128.

Franco E, Ferenczy A. Is HPV testing with cytological triage a more logical approach in cervical cancer screening?*The Lancet Oncology* 2006;7(7):527–529.

Gunnell AS, Tran TN, Torrång A, Dickman PW, Sparén P, Palmgren J, Ylitalo N. Synergy between Cigarette Smoking and Human Papillomavirus Type 16 in Cervical Cancer *in situ* Development. *Cancer Epidemiol Biomarkers Prev* 2006;15; 2141–2147.

Harris TG, Kulasingam SL, Kiviat NB, Mao C, Agoff SN, Feng Q, Koutsky LA.. Cigarette Smoking, Oncogenic Human Papillomavirus, Ki-67 Antigen, and Cervical Intraepithelial Neoplasia.*Am J Epidemiol* 2004; 159(9):834–842.

Hawkes AP, Kronenberger CB, MacKenzie TD, et al. Cervical Cancer Screening. *Am J Prev Med* 1996;12(5):342–344.

Hildesheim A, Hadjimichael O, Schwartz PE, et al. Risk Factors for Rapid-Onset Cervical Cancer. *Am J Obstet Gynecol* 1999;180 (3 Pt 1):571–577. .

International Agency for Research on Cancer (IARC). *Handbooks of Cancer Prevention: Cervix Cancer Screening*, vol. 10. Lyon, France: IARC; 2005.

Kulasingam SL, Hughes JP, Kiviat NB, et al. Evaluation of Human Papillomavirus Testing in Primary Screening for Cervical Abnormalities: Comparison of Sensitivity, Specificity, and Frequency of Referral. *JAMA* 2002;288(14):1749–1757.

Manhart LE, Holmes KK, Koutsky LA, et al. Human Papillomavirus Infection among Sexually Active Young Women in the United States: Implications for Developing a Vaccination Strategy. *Sex Transm Dis* 2006;33:502–508.

Martin-Hirsch P, Lilford R, Jarvis G, Kitchener HC. Efficacy of Cervical-Smear Collection Devices: A Systematic Review and Meta-Analysis. *Lancet* 1999;354 (9192):1763–1770.

Mayo Clinic. Pap Smear: Screening Test for Cervical Cancer. http://mayoclinic.com/. Accessed March 2008.

Mayrand MH, Duarte-Franco E, Rodrigues I, et al. DNA versus Papanicolaou Screening Tests for Cervical Cancer. *NEJM* 2007; 357(16):1579–1588.

Memorial Sloan-Kettering. Risk Factors for Cervical Cancer. http://www.mskcc.org/mskcc/html/13116.cfm. Accessed April 2008.

Memorial Sloan-Kettering Cancer Center. Cervical Cancer Screening Guidelines. http://www.mskcc.org/mskcc/html/65284.cfm. Accessed April 2008.

Moreno V, Bosch FX, Muñoz N, et al. Effect of oral contraceptives on risk of cervical cancer in women with human papillomavirus infection: the IARC multicentric case-control study. *Lancet* 2002;359(9312):1085

Muñoz N, Franceschi S, Bosetti C, et al. Role of Parity and Human Papillomavirus in Cervical Cancer: The IARC Multicentric Case-Control Study. *Lancet* 2002;359 (9312):1093.

Naucler P, Ryd W, Törnberg S, Strand A, Wadell G, Elfgren K, Rådberg T, Strander B, Forslund O, Hansson BG, Rylander E, and Dillner J. Human Papillomavirus and Papanicolaou Tests to Screen for Cervical Cancer. *NEJM* 357(16):1579–1588.

Palefsky J, M.D. What Your Doctor May Not Tell You About, HPV and Abnormal Pap Smears. New York: Warner Books Inc; 2002

Queensland Association for Healthy Communities. Lesbian Health, Looking After Your Cervix: HPV and Pap Smears. www.qahc.org.au/. Accessed April 2008.

Ries L, Harkins D, Krapcho M, et al. *SEER Cancer Statistics Review, 1975–2003*. Bethesda, MD: National Cancer Institute; 2006.

Ronco G, Segnan N. HPV Testing for Primary Cervical Cancer Screening. *Lancet* 2007;370(9601):1740–1742.

Samoff E, Koumans EH, Markowitz LE, et al. Association of Chlamydia Trachomatis with Persistence of High-Risk Types of Human Papillomavirus in a Cohort of Female Adolescents. *Am J Epidemiol* 2005;162(7):668–675.

Sawaya GF, Kerlikowske K, Lee NC, Gildengorin G, Washington AE. Frequency of Cervical Smear Abnormalities within 3 Years of Normal Cytology. *Obstet Gynecol* 2000;96 (2):219–23.

Smith JS, Green J, de Gonzalez, AB, et al. Cervical Cancer and Use of Hormonal Contraceptives: A Systematic Review. *Lancet* 2003;361(9364):1159.

Smith RA, Cokkinides V, von Eschenbach AC, et al. American Cancer Society Guideline for the Early Detection of Cervical Neoplasia and Cancer. *CA Cancer J Clin* 2002;52(1):8–22.

Soost HJ, Lange HJ, Lehmacher W, Ruffing-Kullman B. The Validation of Cervical Cytology. Sensitivity, Specificity and Predictive Values. *Acta Cytol* 1991;35:8–14.

Szarewski A, Jarvis MJ. Effect of Smoking Cessation on Cervical Lesion Size. *Lancet* 1996;347(9006):941.

Trimble CL, Genkinger JM, Burke AE, et al. Active and Passive Cigarette Smoking and the Risk of Cervical Neoplasia. *Obstet Gynecol* 2005;105:174–181.

Trottier H, Franco EL. The Epidemiology of Genital Human Papillomavirus Infection. *Vaccine* 2006;24:1–15.

Vermund SH, Bhatta MP. Papillomavirus Infections. In: Cohen J, Powderly WG, eds. *Infectious Diseases*, 2nd ed. New York: Mosby, An Imprint of Elsevier; 2004.

*Web*MD. Human Papillomavirus (HPV) test. http://www.webmd.com/sexual-conditions/hpv-genital-warts/human-papillomavirus-hpv-test. Accessed April 2008.

Winer RL, Lee SK, Hughes JP, Adam DE, Kiviat NB, Koutsky LA. Genital Human Papillomavirus Infection: Incidence and Risk Factors in a Cohort of Female University Students. *Am J Epidemiol* 2003;157:218–26.

CHAPTER 4: CANCER, WARTS, AND HPV: FROM HEAD AND NECK LESIONS TO CERVICAL, PENILE, AND ANAL DISEASES

ACOG Committee Opinion #301: Sexually transmitted diseases in adolescents. *Obstet Gynecol* 2004;104(4):891–898.

ACOG Treatment Recommendations for Cytologic and Histologic Abnormalities in Adolescents and Adults.*Obstet Gynecol* 2006;107:963–968.

American Academy of Dermatology. Genital warts. http://www.aad.org/public/publications/pamphlets/viral_genital.html. Accessed April 2008.

American Cancer Society (ACS). What Every Woman Should Know about Cervical Cancer and the Human Papilloma Virus. http://www.cancer.org/docroot/home/index.asp. Accessed April 2008.

American Social Health Association. National HPV and Cervical Cancer Prevention Resource Center. http://www.ashastd.org/hpv/hpv_overview.cfm. Accessed April 2008.

Baseman JG, Koutsky LA. The epidemiology of Human Papillomavirus Infections. *J Clin Virol* 2005;32 Suppl 1:S16–24.

Benard VB, Coughlin SS, Thompson T, Richardson LC. Cervical Cancer Incidence in the United States by Area of Residence, 1998–2001. *The American College of Obstetricians and Gynecologists.* 2007 September;110(3):681–686.

Canavan TP, Cohen D. Vulvar Cancer. *American Family Physician* 2002;66(7): 1269–74.

Centers for Disease Control and Prevention (CDC). Genital HPV infection—CDC Fact Sheet. Genital HPV Infection.http://www.cdc.gov/std/HPV/STDFact-HPV.htm. Accessed April 2008.

Chesson HW, Blandford JM, Gift TL, et al. The Estimated Direct Medical Cost of Sexually Transmitted Diseases among American Youth 2000. *Perspect Sex Reprod Health* 2004;36(1):11–19.

Chuang TY, Perry HO, Kurland LT, Ilstrup DM. Condyloma acuminatum in Rochester, Minn., 1950–1978. I. Epidemiology and clinical features. *Arch Dermatol* 1984;120:469–75.

Clifford GM, Smith JS, Plummer M, et al. Human Papillomavirus Types in Invasive Cervical Cancer Worldwide: a Meta-Analysis. *Br J Cancer* 2003;88:63–73.

Coronado GD, Thompson B, Koepsell TD, et al. Use of Pap Test among Hispanics and non-Hispanic Whites in a Rural Setting. *Prev Med* 2004;38:713–722.

Daling JR, Madeleine MM, Schwartz SM, et al. A Population-Based Study of Squamous Cell Vaginal Cancer: HPV and Cofactors. *Gynecol Oncol* 2002;84:263–70.

FIGO System of Cervical Cancer Staging. http://www.figo.org/docs/staging_booklet.pdf. Accessed April 2008.

Fleurence RL, Dixon JM, Milanova TF, Beusterien KM. Review of the Economic and Quality-of-Life Burden of Cervical Human Papillomavirus Disease. *Am J Obstet Gynecol* 2007;196(3).

Gall, SA. Female Genital Warts: Global Trends and Treatments. *Infect Dis Obstet Gynecol* 2001;9:149–154.

Giuliano AR, Papenfuss M, Schneider A, Nour M, Hatch K. Risk Factors for High-Risk Type Human Papillomavirus Infection among Mexican-American Women. *Cancer Epidemiol Biomarkers Prev* 1999;8:615–620.

Greer CE, Wheeler CM, Ladner MB, et al. Human Papillomavirus (HPV) Type Distribution and Serological Response to HPV Type 6 Virus-like Particles in Patients with Genital Warts. *J Clin Microbiol* 1995;33:2058–63.

Haber G, Malow RM, Zimet GD. The HPV Vaccine Mandate Controversy. *Journal of Pediatric and Adolescent Gynecology* 2007;20(6):325–331.

Hall HI, Jamison PM, Coughlin SS. Breast and Cervical Cancer Mortality in the Mississippi Delta, 1979–1998. *South Med J* 2004;97:264–272.

Hopenhayn C, Bush H, Christian A, Shelton BJ. Comparative Analysis of Invasive Cervical Cancer Incidence Rates in Three Appalachian States.*Preventive Medicine* 2005;41(5-6):859–864.

Howell EA, Chen YT, Concato J. Differences in Cervical Cancer Mortality Among Black and White Women. *The American College of Obstetricians and Gynecologists.* 1999;94(4):509–515.

Insinga RP, Glass AG, Rush BB. The Healthcare Costs of Cervical Human Papillomavirus-Related Disease. *Am J Obstet Gynecol* 2004;191(1):114–120.

Judson PL, Habermann EB, Baxter NN, Durham SB, Virnig BA. Trends in the Incidence of Invasive and in situ Vulvar Carcinoma. *Obstet Gynecol* 2006;107: 1018–22.

Kodner, CM, Nasraty S. Management of Genital Warts. *American Family Physician* 2004;70:335–42, 2345–6.

Koutsky L. Epidemiology of Genital Human Papillomavirus Infection. *Am J Med* 1997;102:3–8.

Lipke MM. An Armamentarium of Wart Treatments. *Clin Med Res* 2006; 4(4): 273–293.

National Cancer Institute. Anal Cancer. http://www.cancer.gov/cancertopics/types/anal. Accessed April 2008.

National Cancer Institute. Cervical Cancer. http://www.cancer.gov/cancertopics/types/cervical. Accessed April 2008.

National Cancer Institute. Oropharyngeal Cancer. http://www.cancer.gov/cancertopics/hpv-oropharyngeal-cancer0507. Accessed April 2008.

National Cancer Institute. Vaginal Cancer. http://www.cancer.gov/cancertopics/types/vaginal. Accessed April 2008.

National Cancer Institute. Vulvar Cancer. http://www.cancer.gov/cancertopics/types/vulvar. Accessed April 2008.

National Institute of Allergies and Infectious Diseases. Human Pappilomavirus and Genital Warts. http://www3.niaid.nih.gov/healthscience/healthtopics/human_papillomavirus/. Accessed April 2008.

Palefsky J. What Your Doctor May Not Tell You About, HPV and Abnormal Pap Smears. New York: Warner Books Inc; 2002.

Parkin M, Bray F. The Burden of HPV Related Cancers. *Vaccine* 2006; 24(S3): S11–S25.

Porterfield DS, Dutton G, Gizlice Z. Cervical Cancer in North Carolina. Incidence, Mortality and Risk Factors. *North Carolina Medical Journal* 2003; 64: 11–7.

Saraiya M. Incidence Rates for Invasive Cervical Cancer by Age (in Years) and Race or Ethnicity, United States 1988–2002. *Obstet Gynecol* 2007; 109(2Pt1):360–370.

Schiffman M, Castle PE. The Promise of Global Cervical-Cancer Prevention. *NEJM* 2005;353(20):2101–2104.

Seeff LC, McKenna MT. Cervical Cancer Mortality among Foreign-Born Women Living in the United States, 1985 to 1996. *Cancer Detection and Prevention* 2004;27(3):203–208.

Solomon D, Breen N, McNeel T. Cervical Cancer Screening Rates in the United States and the Potential Impact of Implementation of Screening Guidelines. *CA Cancer J Clin* 2007; 57(2):105–11.

Soper D. Reducing the Health Burden of HPV Infection Through Vaccination. *Infect Dis Obstet Gynecol* 2006; published online, doi: 10.1155/IDOG/2006/83084.

Tirol JA, Meissner HI, Kobrin S, Chollette V. What Do Women in the U.S. Know about Human Papillomavirus and Cervical Cancer? *Cancer Epidemiol Biomarkers Prev* 2007;16, 288–294.

U.S. Cancer Statistics Working Group. *United States Cancer Statistics: 2004 Incidence and Mortality.* Atlanta (GA): Department of Health and Human Services, Centers for Disease Control and Prevention, and National Cancer Institute; 2007.

Wilkinson EJ. ASCCP Practice Guidelines Management Guidelines for the Follow-up of Cytology Interpreted as Benign Cellular Changes on Papanicolaou Smear of the Cervix or Vagina. *Journal of Lower Genital Tract Disease* 2000; 4(2):93.

Yabroff KR, Lawrence WF, King JC, et al. Geographic Disparities in Cervical Cancer Mortality: What Are the Roles of Risk Factor Prevalence, Screening, and Use of Recommended Treatment? *J Rural Health* 2005;21:149–157.

CHAPTER 5: EMOTIONAL ASPECTS AND PREVENTION OF HPV: SHAME, BLAME, AND ABSENCE OF CURE

Badia X, Colombo JA, Lara N, et al. Combination of Qualitative and Quantitative Methods for Developing a New Health Related Quality of Life Measure for Patients with Anogenital Warts. *Health and Quality of Life Outcomes* 2005;3:24.

Bosch FX, Lorincz A, Munoz N, et al. The Causal Relation between Human Papillomavirus and Cervical Cancer. *J Clin Pathol* 2002;55:244–265.

Campion M, Brown JR, McCance DJ, et al., Psychosexual Trauma of an Abnormal Pap Smear, *BJOG* 1988;95(2):175–181.

Centers for Disease Control (CDC). Incidence of Pap Test Abnormalities with 3 Years of a Normal Pap Test—1991–1998. *Mortality and Morbidity Weekly Report* 2000; 49(44):1001–1004.

Clarke P, Ebel C, Catotti DN, Stewart S. The Psychological Impact of Human Papillomavirus Infection: Implications for Health Care Providers. *Int J STD and AIDS* 1996; 7(3):197–200.

Cunningham SD, Kerrigan D, Pillay KB, et al. Understanding the Role of Perceived Severity in STD-Related Care-Seeking Delays. *J Adolesc Health* 2005;37:69–74.

Cunningham SD, Tschann J, Gurvey JE, et al. Attitudes about sexual disclosure and perceptions of stigma and shame. *Sexually Transm Infect* 2002;78:334–338.

Duncan B, Hart G, Scoular A, et al. Qualitative Analysis of Psychosocial Impact of Diagnosis of Chlamydia trachomatis: Implications for Screening. *BMJ* 2001;322:195–199.

Filiberti A, Tamburini M, Stefanon B, et al. Psychological Aspects of Genital Human Papillomavirus Infection: A Preliminary Report. *J Psychosom Obstet Gynaecol* 1993 June;14(2):145–152.

Fortenberry JD, McFarlane M, Bleakley A, et al. Relationships of Stigma and Shame to Gonorrhea and HIV Screening. *Am J Public Health* 2002;92:378–381.

Guy H. Survey Shows How We Live with HPV, *HPV News* 1993;3(2):1 and 4–8.

Kerr Y, Williams M, Stoner B. Physicians Knowledge about Human Papillomavirus in Relationship to External Genital warts and Cervical Cancer. National STD Prevention Conference, Milwaukee, December 2000.

Linnehan MJE, Groce NE. Psychosocial and Educational Services For Female College Students with Genital Human Papillomavirus Infection. *Family Planning Perspectives* 1999;31(3):137–141.

Linnehan MJE, Groce NE. Counseling and Educational Interventions for Women with Genital Human Papillomavirus Infection. *AIDS Patient Care and STDs* 2000;14(8):439–445. doi: 10.1089/108729100416650.

Maissi E, Marteau TM, Hankins M, et al. The Psychological Impact of Human Papillomavirus Testing in Women with Borderline or Mildly Dyskaryoticcervical Smear Test Results: 6-Month Follow-up. *Br J Cancer* 2005;92:990–4.

Maissi E, Marteau TM, Hankins M, Moss S, Legood R, Gray A. Psychological Impact of Human Papillomavirus Testing in Women with Borderline or Mildly Dyskaryotic Cervical Smear Test Results: Cross Sectional Questionnaire Study *BMJ* 2004 29 May;328:1293.

Mast TC, Gupta S, Coplan P. Measuring HPV Related Quality of life—Challenges for the Future. 19th International Papillomavirus Conference, Brazil. September 2001.

McCaffery K, Waller J, Forrest S, et al. Testing Positive for Human Papillomavirus in Routine Cervical Screening: examination of Psychosocial Impact. *BJOG* 2004;111:1437–1443.

McCaffery K, Waller J, Nazroo J, et al. Social and Psychological Impact of HPV Testing in Cervical Screening: a Qualitative Study. *Sexually Transm Infect* 2006;82:169–74.

Newton DC, Newtown C, McCabe MP. The Impact of Stigma on Couples Managing a Sexually Transmitted Infection. *Sexual & Relationship Therapy* 2005; 20(1):51–63.

Waller J, Marlow LAV, Wardle J. The Association between Knowledge of HPV and Feelings of Stigma, Shame and Anxiety. *Sexually Transm Infect* 2007;83:155–159.

Waller J, McCaffery K, Forrest S, et al. Awareness of Human Papillomavirus among Women Attending a Well Woman Clinic. *Sexually Transm Infect* 2003;79:320.

Wyand F. Emotional Solitaire. What you Need to Know About Cervical Cancer Prevention and Genital Warts. HPV e- news, June 2007. www.ashastd.org/learn/learn_hpv_warts_sup.cfm. Accessed April 2008.

Chapter 6: The New HPV Vaccines: History, Recommendations, and Limitations

Abou-Daoud KT. Epidemiology of Carcinoma of the Cervix Uteri in Lebanese Christians and Moslems. *Cancer* 1967;20:1706–1714.

Adams M, Jasani B, Fiander A. Human Papilloma Virus (HPV) Prophylactic Vaccination: Challenges for Public Health and Implications for Screening. *Vaccine* 2007;25(16):3007–30013.

Ault KA, Giuliano AR, Edwards RP, et al. A Phase I Study to Evaluate a Human Papillomavirus (HPV) Type 18 L1 VLP Vaccine. *Vaccine* 2004;22(23-24):3004–3007.

Baden LR, Curfman GD, Morrissey S, Drazen JM. Human Papillomavirus Vaccine—Opportunity and Challenge. *NEJM* 2007;356(19):1990–1991.

Braithwaite J. Excess of Salt in the Diet: a Probable Factor in the Causation of Cancer. *Lancet* 1901;ii:1578–1580.

Capell K, Barrett A. A Vaccine Every Woman Should Take. *Business Week*. November 29,2004. Available online at http://www.businessweek.com/magazine/content/04_48/b3910080_mz054.htm. Accessed April 2008.

Centers for Disease Control (CDC). HPV: Gardasil and GBS. CDC/Office of the Chief Science Office/Immunization Safety Office, August 15, 2007. http://www.cdc.gov/vaccines/vpd-vac/hpv/downloads/hpv-gardasil-gbs.pdf. Accessed April 2008.

Cervarix Summary of Product Characteristics. Therapeutic Goods Association, Australia. http://www.medicalnewstoday.com/articles/75783.php. Accessed April 2008.

Chan JK, Berek JS. Impact of the Human Papilloma Vaccine on Cervical Cancer. *J Clin Oncol* 2007;25(20):2975–2982.

Cohen J. High Hopes and Dilemmas for a Cervical Cancer Vaccine, Sciencemag.org; April 29, 2005;308(5722):618–621.

Conversation with the Man Behind the HPV Vaccine. Georgetown University Medical Center, Office of Communications. October 24, 2006 (Talk given by Dr. Richard Schlegel).

Davis K, Dickman ED, Ferris D, Dias JK. Human Papillomavirus Vaccine Acceptability among Parents of 10- to 15-Year-Old Adolescents. *J Low Genit Tract Dis* 2004;8:188–194.

Dell DL, Chen H, Ahmad F, Stewart DE. Knowledge about Human Papillomavirus among Adolescents. *Obstet Gynecol* 2000;96:653–656.

Dunn JE, Buell P. Association of Cervical Cancer with Circumcision of Sexual Partner. *J Natl Cancer Inst* 1959;22:746–749.

Dunne E. HPV Vaccine Update. Division of STD Prevention, CDC, ACHA Meeting May 2007.

Dunne E, Unger E, et al. Prevalence of HPV Infection Among Females in the United States. *JAMA* 2007;297:813–819.

Gardasil Prescribing Information. http://www.gardasil.com/downloads/gardasil_pi.pdf.

Garland SM, Hernandez-Avila M, Wheeler CM, et al. (FUTURE I Investigators). Quadrivalent Vaccine against Human Papillomavirus to Prevent High-Grade Cervical Lesions. *N Engl J Med* 2007;356:1915–1927.

Garland SM, Hernandez-Avila M, Wheeler CM, et al., for the Females United to Unilaterally Reduce Endo/Ectocervical Disease (FUTURE) I Investigators. Quadrivalent Vaccine against Human Papillomavirus to Prevent Anogenital Diseases.*N Engl J Med* 2007; 356(19):1928–1943.

Goldie SJ, Kohli M, Grima D, et al. Projected Clinical Benefits and Cost-Effectiveness of a Human Papillomavirus 16/18 Vaccine. *J Natl Cancer Inst* 2004;96:604–615.

Human Papillomavirus, ACOG Practice Bulletin No. 61. *Obstet Gynecol* 2005;105:905–18.

Hymel PA. Decreasing Risk: Impact of HPV Vaccination on Outcomes. *Am J Managed Care* 2006;12:S473–S483.

Ireland C. A Cancer Vaccine Is Born. *Rochester Review*; University of Rochester. 2006;68(3)

Kaylin J. The Virus Behind the Cancer. *Yale Medicine* Spring 2006.

Kulasingam SL, Myers ER. Potential Health and Economic Impact of Adding a Human Papillomavirus Vaccine to Screening Programs. *JAMA* 2003;290:781–789

Lambert EC. College Students' Knowledge of Human Papillomavirus and Effectiveness of a Brief Educational Intervention. *J Am Board Fam Pract* 2001; 14:178–183. .

Mao C, Koutsky LA, Ault KA, et al. Efficacy of Human Papillomavirus-16 Vaccine to Prevent cervical Intraepithelial Neoplasia: A randomized Controlled Trial. *Obstet Gynecol* 2006;107:18–27.

Markowitz LE, Dunne EF, Saraiya M, Lawson HW, Chesson H, Unger ER. Quadrivalent Human Papillomavirus Vaccine—Recommendations of the Advisory Committee on Immunization Practices (ACIP), Centers for Disease Control.

McIntyre P. Finding the Viral Link—The Story of Harald zur Hausen. *Cancer World* July-August 2005. http://www.cancerworld.org/CancerWorld/getStaticModFile.aspx?id=717. Accessed April 2008.

McNeil DG. How a Vaccine Search Ended in Triumph. *The New York Times.* August 29, 2006. http://www.nytimes.com/2006/08/29/health/29hpv.html. Accessed April 2008.

McNeil DG. New Cervical Cancer Vaccine Highly Promising but Questions Remain. *Harvard Women's Health Watch* 2007;14(12):1–3. http://web.ebscohost.com .monstera.cc.columbia.edu:2048/ehost/pdf?vid=4&hid=113&sid=f26cecb7-cc3e-4fff-8c05-b5799663bcce%40sessionmgr108. Accessed April 2008.

Middleman AB. Immunization Update: Pertussis, Meningoccocus, and Human Papillomavirus. *Adolescent Medicine Clinics*2006;17(3):547–563.

National Cancer Institute. Human Papillomavirus Vaccines: Questions and Answers Fact Sheet. http://www.cancer.gov/cancertopics/factsheet/risk/HPV-vaccine. Accessed April 2008.

National Institutes of Health (NIH)—Office of Technology Transfer. NIH Technology Licensed to Merck for HPV Vaccine. September 18, 2006. Available online at http://www.ott.nih.gov/current_issues/issues-ended-09-18-2006.html. Accessed May 2008.

New York State Department of Health. *Questions and Answers about HPV vaccine.* Available online at http://www.health.state.ny.us/prevention/immunization/human_papillomavirus/index.htm. Accessed May 2008.

Prescribing information for GARDASIL. Whitehouse Station (NJ): Merck & Co., Inc.; 2006.

Rawls WE, Tompkins WA, Figueroa ME, Melnick JL. Herpesvirus Type 2: Association with Carcinoma of the Cervix. Science 1968;161:1255–1256.

Roehr B. HPV Vaccine Provides Cross-Protection Against Other Strains. *Medscape Medical News.,* September 20, 2007 (Chicago).

Royston I, Aurelian L. The Association of Genital Herpesvirus with Cervical Atypia and Carcinoma in situ. *Am J Epidemiol* 1970;91:531–538.

Sanders GD, Taira AV. Cost-Effectiveness of a Potential Vaccine for Human Papillomavirus. *Emerg Infect Dis* 2003;9:37–48.

Saslow D, Castle PE, Cox TJ, et al American Cancer Society Guideline for Human Papillomavirus (HPV) Vaccine Use to Prevent Cervical Cancer and Its Precursors.*CA Cancer J Clin* 2007;57;7–28.

Sawaya GF, Smith-McCune K. HPV Vaccination–More Answers, More Questions. *NEJM* 2007;356(19):1991–1993.

Schiller JT, Davies P. Delivering on the Promise: HPV Vaccines and Cervical Cancer. *Nature Rev Microbiology.* 2004;2(4):343–347.

Schiller JT, Lowy DR. Papillomavirus-like Particles and HPV Vaccine Development. *Seminars in Cancer Biology* 1996;7(6):373–382.

Schwarz TF. Human Papillomavirus-16/18 Candidate Vaccine Adjuvanted with AS04 and its Impact on the Incidence of Cervical Cancer. Expert Rev. *Obstet Gynecol* 2007;2(3),293–303.

Soper D. Reducing the Health Burden of HPV Infection Through Vaccination. *Infect Dis Obstet Gynecol* 2006; published online, doi: 10.1155/IDOG/2006/83084.

Stanley M, Lowy DR, Frazer I. Prophylactic Vaccines: Underlying Mechanisms. *Vaccine* 2006;24:S106–S113.

Statement form the National Cancer Institute on FDA Approval of the HPV Vaccine. http://www.cancer.gov/newscenter/pressreleases/HPVStatement. Accessed April 2008.

Steinbrook R. The Potential of Human Papillomavirus Vaccines. *NEJM* 2006;354 (11):1109–1112.

Vaccine Guide: Risks and Benefits for Children and Adults. Randall Neustaedter. 2002.

Villa LL, Costa RL, Petta CA, et al. Prophylactic Quadrivalent Human Papillomavirus (types 6, 11, 16, and 18) L1 Viruslike Particle Vaccine in Young Women: A Randomised Double Blind Placebo-Controlled Multicentre Phase II Efficacy Trial. *The Lancet Oncology* 2005;6(5):271–278.

Villa LL, Costa RL, Petta CA, et al. Duration of Immunity—High Sustained Efficacy of a Prophylactic Quadrivalent Human Papillomavirus Types 6/11/16/18 L1 Virus-like Particle Vaccine through 5 Years of Follow-up. *Br J Cancer* 2006;95:1459–1466.

Waller J, McCaffery K, Forrest S, et al. Awareness of Human Papillomavirus among Women Attending a Well Woman Clinic. *Sexually Transm Infect* 2003;79:320–322. .

World Health Organization (WHO). Initiative for Vaccine Research. http://www.who.int/vaccine_research/en/. Accessed April 2008.

Chapter 7: HPV Vaccines for Males: The Unsolved Half of the Equation

Aguilar LV, Lazcano-Ponce E, Vaccarella S, et al. Human Papillomavirus in Men: Comparison of Different Genital Sites. *Sexually Transm Infect* 2006;82:31–33.

Allday E. Doctors Want Pap Test for Gay Men. *San Francisco Chronicle.* April 21, 2007. Found online at http://www.sfgate.com/cgi-bin/article.cgi?f=/c/a/2007/04/21/BAGUNPCQN61.DTL. Accessed June 2008.

American Cancer Society (ACS). Cancer Facts and Figures 2006. http://www.cancer.org/downloads/STT/CAFF2006PWSecured.pdf. Accessed April 2008.

American Social Health Association. National HPV and Cervical Cancer Prevention Resource Center. Learn About HPV: What Women Should Know. http://www.ashastd.org/hpv/hpv_learn_women.cfm. Accessed April 2008.

Baldwin, et al. Condom Use and Other Factors Affecting Penile HPV Detection in Men. *STD's* 2004;31(10):601–607

Blacklow NR. Condom Use Reduces Risk for HPV Infection in Women. *Journal Watch Infect Diseases* July 12, 2006:2.

Bosch FX, Castellsague X, Munoz N, et al. Male Sexual Behavior and Human Papillomavirus DNA: Key Risk Factors for Cervical Cancer in Spain. *J Natl Cancer Inst* 1996;88:1060–1067.

Castellsagué X, Bosch FX, Muñoz N, et al. Male Circumcision, Penile Human Papillomavirus Infection, and Cervical Cancer in Female Partners. *NEJM* 2002;346 (15);1105–1112.

Centers for Disease Control and Prevention (CDC). US Cancer Statistics Working Group. *United States Cancer Statistics: 2003. Incidence and Mortality.* Atlanta, GA: U.S. Department of Health and Human Services, CDC, and the National Cancer Institute. 2005. Available at http://www.cdc.gov/uscs. Accessed May 2008.

Centers for Disease Control and Prevention (CDC). HPV and Men—CDC Fact Sheet. Page last reviewed August 14, 2007. http://www.cdc.gov/STD/hpv/STDFact-HPV-and-men.htm. Accessed April 2008.

Chin-Hong PV, Vittinghoff E, Cranston RD, et al. Age-Specific Prevalence of Anal Human Papillomavirus Infection in HIV-Negative Sexually Active Men Who Have Sex with Men: The EXPLORE Study. *J Infect Dis* December 15,2004;190 (12):2070–2076

Daling JR, Madeleine MM, Johnson LG, et al. Penile Cancer: Importance of Circumcision, Human Papillomavirus and Smoking in situ and Invasive Disease. *Int J Cancer* 2005;116(4):606–616.

D'Souza G, Kreimer AR, Viscidi R, et al. Case-Control Study of Human Papillomavirus and Oropharyngeal Cancer. *NEJM*2007;356(19):1944–1956.

Dunne EF, Nielson CM, Stone KM, Markowitz LE, Giuliano AR. Prevalence of HPV Infections among Men; Systemic Review of the Literature. *J Infect Dis* 2006;194:1044–1057.

El-Hout Y, Khauli RB. The Case for Routine Circumcision. *Journal of Men's Health & Gender* September 2007;4(3): 300–305.

Frega A, French D, Pace S, et al. Prevalence of Acetowhite Areas in Male Partners of Women Affected by HPV and Squamous Intra-epithelial Lesions (SIL) and Their Prognostic Significance. A Multicenter Study. *J Lower Genital Tract Disease* 2007 11(2):130.

Garland SM, Hernandez-Avila M, Wheeler CM, et al, for the Females United to Unilaterally Reduce Endo/Ectocervical Disease (FUTURE) I Investigators. Quadrivalent Vaccine against Human Papillomavirus to Prevent Anogenital Diseases.*NEJM*2007;356(19):1928–1943.

Gearheart PA. Human Papillomavirus. Department of Obstetrics and Gynecology, Pennsylvania Hospital. http://www.emedicine.com/med/TOPIC1037.HTM. Accessed April 2008.

Geipert N.Vaccinating Men for HPV: New Strategy for Preventing Cervical Cancer in Women? *JNCI J Natl Cancer Inst*2005;97(9):630–631.

Giuliano AR, Nielson CM, Flores R, et al. The Optimal Anatomic Sites for Sampling Heterosexual Men for Human Papillomavirus (HPV) Detection: The HPV Detectionin Men Study. *J Infect Dis* 2007 October 15:196(8): 1146–1152.

Giuliano AR, Papenfuss M, Schneder A, Nour M, Hatch M. Risk Factors for High-Risk Type Human Papillomavirus Infection among Mexican-American Women. *Cancer Epidemiol Biomarkers Prev* 1999;8:615–620.

Goodman MT, Hernandez BY, Shvetsov YB. Demographic and Pathologic Differences in the Incidence of Invasive Penile Cancer in the United States, 1995–2003. *Cancer Epidemiol Biomarkers Prev* 2007;16;1833–1839.

H. Lee Moffitt Cancer Center & Research Institute. Men's Research Study. http://www.moffitt.org/Site.aspx?spid=F0E006A8BC9A4B86A972CDD9CF599528. Accessed April 2008.

H. Lee Moffitt Cancer Center & Research Institute- HPV Research. http://www.moffitt.org/Site.aspx?spid=F0E006A8BC9A4B86A972CDD9CF599528. Accessed April 2008.

Hans-Olov A, Trichopoulos D. Cervical Cancer and the Elusive Male Factor. *NJEM* 2002;346:1160–1161.

Hirschmann JV. Condoms Still Important in Preventing Human Papillomavirus Infection. *Journal Watch Dermatology.* July 14, 2006: 5-5.

Kaunitz AM. Can Consistent Condom Use Contain HPV? *Journal Watch Women's Health.* July 20, 2006;4-4.

Knight D. Health Care Screening for Men Who Have Sex with Men. *American Family Physician, American Academy of Family Physicians.* 2004;69(19).

Koutsky L, Epidemiology of Genital Human Papillomavirus Infection. *The American Journal of Medicine* 1997;102(5S1):3–8.

Kreimer AR, Clifford GM, Boyle P, and Franceschi S. Human Papillomavirus Types in Head and Neck Squamous Cell Carcinomas Worldwide: A Systematic Review. *Cancer Epidemiol Biomarkers Prev* 2005;14:467–475.

Liang W, Cottler L, Garvin EC, Callahan C, Winer RL, Koutsky LA. Condom Use and the Risk of HPV Infection. *NEJM* 2006;355:1388–1389.

MacLachlan K, Jacobs JR. Male HPV Infection: A Challenge for Diagnosis and Treatment. ACHA 2007 Annual Meeting June 1, 2007, San Antonio, TX.

Manseck A. Prevention of Penile Cancer. Value of the HPV Vaccination and Circumcision. *Urologe A* 2007;46(6):646–50. Abstract in English.

Micali G, Nasca MR, Innocenzi D, Schwartz RA. Penile cancer. *J Am Academy Dermatology* 2006;54(3):369–391.

National HPV Vaccinating Program. Australian Government, Department of Health and Aging. http://www.health.sa.gov.au/pehs/Cervix-screening/hpv-vaccine.htm. Accessed April 2008.

Nielson CM, Flores R, Harris RB, et al. Human Papillomavirus Prevalence and Type Distribution in Male Anogenital Sites.*Cancer Epidemiol Biomarkers Prev* 2007;16;1107–1114.

Nielson CM, Harris RB, Dunne EF, Abrahamsen M, et al. Risk Factors for Anogenital Human Papillomavirus Infection in Men. *J Infect Dis* 2007;196:1137–1145.

Palefsky J. Beyond Cervical Cancer: Other Anogenital Cancers Caused by HPV Infection. http://www.medscape.com/viewarticle/549567_1. Accessed April 2008.

Palefsky JM, Holly EA, Efirdc JT, Da Costa M, Jay N, B JM, Darragh TM. Anal Intraepithelial Neoplasia in the Highly Active Antiretroviral Therapy Era among HIV-Positive Men Who Have Sex with Men. *AIDS* 2005;19(13): 1407–1414 .

Partridge JM, Koutsky LA. Genital Human Papillomavirus Infection in Men. *The Lancet Infectious Diseases* 2006;6(1):21–31.

Pirani C. Cervical Jabs for Boys. *The Australian.* News from Australia's National Newspaper, September 13, 2007. Available online at www.theaustralian.news.com.au/story/0,20867,21108386-23289,00.html. Accessed May 2008.

Ryan DP, Compton CC, Mayer RJ. Carcinoma of the Anal Canal. 2000;342(11): 792–800.

Schottenfeld D, Winawer S. Cancers of the Large Intestine. In: Schottenfeld D, Fraumeni J., eds. *Cancer Epidemiology and Prevention.* New York: Oxford University Press; 1996:813–840.

Sturgis EM, Cinciripini PM. Trends in Head and Neck Cancer Incidence in Relation to Smoking Prevalence—An Emerging Epidemic of Human Papillomavirus-Associated Cancers? *Cancer* 2007;110(7):1429–1435.

Syrjänen S .Human Papillomaviruses in Head and Neck Carcinomas. *NEJM* 2007;356(19):1993–1995.

US Cancer Statistics Working Group. *United States Cancer Statistics: 2004. Incidence and Mortality.* Atlanta, GA: US Department of Health and Human Services, CDC and the National Cancer Institute; 2005. Available online at http://apps.nccd.cdc.gov/uscs/. Accessed May 2008.

Weaver BA, Feng Q, Holmes KK, et al. Evaluation of Genital Sites and Sampling Techniques for Detection of Human Papillomavirus DNA in Men. *J Infect Dis* 2004;15:189.

Weintrub PS. Condoms Prevent the Transmission of Human Papillomavirus. *Journal Watch Pediatrics.* July 12, 2006: 2-2.

What's New in the Other General Journals. *BMJ* 333: 37–38.

Winer RL, Hughes JP, Feng Q, et al. Condom Use and the Risk of Genital Human Papillomavirus Infection in Young Women. *NEJM* 2006;354(25): 2645–2654

Zuger A. Condoms Reduce HPV Acquisition in Heterosexual Women. *Journal Watch General.* June 30, 2006: 7.

CHAPTER 8: FAQ's on HPV and the Vaccines: Excerpts from a University Town Hall Meeting

Centers for Disease Control and Prevention (CDC). *2002 National Survey of Family Growth.* Available online at http://www.cdc.gov/nchs/nsfg.htm. Accessed May 2008.

Gardasil Prescribing Information. http://www.gardasil.com/downloads/gardasil _pi.pdf.

Greer CE, Wheeler CM, Ladner MB, et al. Human Papillomavirus (HPV) Type Distribution and Serological Response to HPV Type 6 Virus-like Particles in Patients with Genital Warts. *J Clin Microbiol* 1995;33:2058–2063.

Gunnell AS, Tran TN, Torrång A, et al. Synergy between Cigarette Smoking and Human Papillomavirus Type 16 in Cervical Cancer In situ Development. *Cancer Epidemiol Biomarkers Prev* 2006;15; 2141–2147.

Manhart LE, Holmes KK, Koutsky LA, et al. Human Papillomavirus Infection among Sexually Active Young Women in the United States: Implications for Developing a Vaccination Strategy. *Sex Transm Dis* 2006;33:502–8.

Moreno V, Bosch FX, Muñoz N, et al. Effect of Oral Contraceptives on Risk of Cervical Cancer in Women with Human Papillomavirus Infection: The IARC Multicentric Case-Control Study. *Lancet* 2002;359(9312):1085.

Schottenfeld D, Winawer S. Cancers of the Large Intestine. In: Schottenfeld D, Fraumeni J, eds. *Cancer Epidemiology and Prevention.* New York: Oxford University Press; 1996:813–840.

Villa LL, Costa RL, Petta CA, et al. High Sustained Efficacy of a Prophylactic Quadrivalent Human Papillomavirus Types 6/11/16/18 L1 Virus-like Particle Vaccine through 5 Years of Follow-up. *Br J Cancer* 2006;95:1459–66.

Walboomers JM, Jacobs MV, Manos MM, et al. Human Papillomavirus Is a Necessary Cause of Invasive Cervical Cancer Worldwide. *J Pathol* 1999;189:12–19.

Weinstock H, Berman S, Cates W Jr. Sexually Transmitted Diseases among American Youth: Incidence and Prevalence Estimates, 2000. *Perspect Sex Reprod Health* 2004;36:6–10.

Winer RL, Hughes JP, Feng Q, et al. Condom Use and the Risk of Genital Human Papillomavirus Infection in Young Women. *NJEM* 2006;354(25):2645–2654.

Chapter 9: Parent's Dilemma to Vaccinate: A Physician Mother's Perspective

Abma JC, Martinez GM, Mosher WD, Dawson BS. Teenagers in the United States: Sexual Activity, Contraceptive Use, and Childbearing, 2002. *Vital and Health Statistics* 2004, Series 23, No. 24.

Albrich WC, BaughmanW, Schmotzer B, Farley MM. Changing Characteristics of Invasive Pneumococcal Disease in Metropolitan Atlanta, Georgia after Introduction of 7-Valent Pnuemococcal Conjugate Vaccine. *Clinical Infectious Disease* 2007; 44:1569–1576.

American College of Obstetricians and Gynecologists. HPV Vaccine. http://www.acog.org/publications/patient_education/bp073.cfm. Accessed April 2008.

American Social Health Association. Frequently asked Questions about Cervical Cancer HPV Vaccine Access in the U.S. http://www.ashastd.org/pdfs/hpv_faq_032007.pdf. Accessed April 2008.

Bonney LE, Lally M, Williams DR, Stein M, Flanigan T. Where to Begin Human Papillomavirus Vaccination?*The Lancet Infectious Diseases*. 2006;6(7):389–390.

Brody JE. HPV Vaccine: Few Risks, Many Benefits. *The New York Times*. May 15, 2007. Available online at http://www.nytimes.com/2007/05/15/health/15brod.html. Accessed May 2008.

Center KJ. Prevenar Vaccination: Review of the Global Data, 2006. *Vaccine*. 2007;22 (16): 3085–3089.

Centers for Disease Control and Prevention (CDC). Trends in Sexual Risk Behaviors among High School Students—United States, 1991–2001. *MMWR* 2002;51: 856–859.

Centers for Disease Control and Prevention (CDC). Youth Risk Behavior Surveillance Summary—United States, 2003, Morbidity and Mortality Weekly Report, May 2004, 53(2).

Chan SSC, Cheung TH, Lo WK, Chung TKH. Women's Attitudes on Human Papillomavirus Vaccinationto Their Daughters. *J Adolesc Health* 2007;41; 204–207.

Charo RA. Politics, Parents, and Prophylaxis—Mandating HPV Vaccination in the United States. *NEJM*. 2007;356(19):1905–1908

Dailard C. Legislating against Arousal: The Growing Divide between Federal Policy and Teenage Sexual Behavior. *Guttmacher Policy Rev* 2006;9:12–16.

Davis K, Dickman ED, Ferris D, Dias JK. Human Papillomavirus Vaccine Accept-
    ability among Parents of 10- to 15-Year-Old Adolescents. *J Low Genit Tract Dis*
    2004;8:188–194.
Dell DL, Chen H, Ahmed F, Stewart DE. Knowledge About Human Papillomavi-
    rus Among Adolescents. *Obstet Gynecol* 2000;96:653–656 .
Dempsey AF, Zimet GD, Davis RL, Koutsky L. Factors That Are Associated with
    Parental Acceptance of Human Papillomavirus Vaccines: A Randomized Interven-
    tion Study of Written Information about HPV. *Pediatrics.* 2006;117(5):1486–1493.
Eaton DK, Kann L, Kinchen S, et al. Youth Risk Behavior Surveillance—United
    States, 2005. *MMWR Surveill Summ.* 2006;55:1–108.
Elbasha E, Dasbach EJ, Insinga RP. Model for Assessing Human Papillomavirus
    Vaccination. *Emerg Infect Dis* 2007;13:29–41.
Esposito S, Bosis S, Pelucchi C, Begliatti E, Rognoni A, et al. Pediatrician Knowl-
    edge and Attitudes Regarding Human Papillomavirus Disease and Its Preven-
    tion. *Vaccine.* 2007;29:6437–6446.
Gostin LO, DeAngenlis C. Mandatory HPV Vaccination—Public Health vs Private
    Wealth.*JAMA.* 2007; 297:1921–1923.
Gust DA, Campbell S, Kennedy A, et al. Parental Concerns and Medical-Seeking
    Behavior after Immunization. *Am J Prev Med* 2006;31:32–35.
Guttmacher Institute. Minors' Access to Contraceptive Services, State Policies in Brief.
    August 1, 2006. Available online at http://www.guttmacher.org/statecenter/
    spibs/spib_MACS.pdf. Accessed August 7, 2006.
Haber G, Malow RM, and Zimet GD. The HPV Vaccine Mandate Controversy.
    Journal of Pediatric and Adolescent Gynecology. 2007;20(6):325–331.
Handsfield HH, with Hoel D. Sex, Science, and Society. A Look at Sexually Trans-
    mitted Diseases. *Postgraduate Medicine.* 1997;101(5):268–275.
Kaiser Family Foundation. National Survey of Adolescents and Young Adults:
    Sexual Health Knowledge, Attitudes and Behaviors. May 2003.
Markowitz LE, Dunne EF, Saraiya M, Lawson HW, Chesson H, Unger ER. Quadri-
    valent Human Papillomavirus Vaccine—Recommendations of the Advisory
    Committee on Immunization Practices (ACIP), Centers for Disease Control.
Mayo Clinic. How Vaccines Work. http://mayoclinic.com/. Accessed March 2008.
Mays RM, Sturm LA, Zimet GD. Parental Perspectives on Vaccinating Children
    against Sexually Transmitted Infections. *Social Science & Medicine.* 2005;58
    (7):1405–1413.
Mosher WD, Chandra A, Jones J. Sexual Behavior and Selected Health Measures:
    Men and Women 15–44 Years of Age, United States, 2002. *Advance Data from
    Vital and Health Statistics,* no 362. Hyattsville, MD: National Center for Health
    Statistics. 2005.
National Foundation for Infectious Diseases. Adolescent Vaccination: Bridging
    from a Strong Childhood Foundation to a Healthy Adulthood. Bethesda, MD:
    National Foundation for Infectious Diseases; 2005. Online at http://www.nfid
    .org/pdf/publications/adolescentvacc.pdf. Accessed April 19, 2007
National Women's Health Network. Vaccines for HPV and Cervical Cancer.
    http://www.nwhn.org/alerts/details.cfm?email_message_id=44. Accessed
    April 2008.
Neinstein LS, Gordon CM, Katzman DK, Rosen DS, Woods ER. *Adolescent Health
    Care: A Practical Guide.*5th ed. Philadelphia: Lippincott Williams and Wilkins;
    2008.

Olshen E, Woods ER, Austin SB, et al. Parental Acceptance of the Human Papillomavirus Vaccine. *J Adolesc Health* 2005;36(2):124.

Olshen E, Woods ER, Austin SB, et al. Parental Acceptance of the Human Papillomavirus Vaccine. *J Adolesc Health* 2005;37:248–251.

Remez L. Oral Sex Among Adolescents: Is It Sex or Is It Abstinence? *Family Planning Perspectives.* Guttmacher Institute. 2000;32(6):298–304.

Rolling out HPV Vaccines Worldwide.*The Lancet.* 2006;367(9528):2034–2034.

Soper D. Reducing the Health Burden of HPV Infection through Vaccination. *Infect Dis Obstet Gynecol* Published online 2006. doi: 10.1155/IDOG/2006/83084.

Stanberry LR, Rosenthal SL. Progress in Vaccines for Sexually Transmitted Diseases. *Infectious Disease Clinics of North America.* 2005;19(2):477–490.

Sugarman SD, J.D. Cases in Vaccine Court—Legal Battles over Vaccines and Autism. *NEJM.* 2007;357(13):1275–1277.

Temte JL. HPV Vaccine: A Cornerstone of Female Health. Editorials. *American Family Physician.* 2007 January 1;75(1):28,20..

Waller J. Mothers' Attitudes towards Preventing Cervical Cancer through Human Papillomavirus Vaccination: A Qualitative Study. *Cancer Epidemiol Biomarkers Prev* 2006 July 1;15(7):1257–1261.

Waller J, McCaffery K, Forrest S, et al. Awareness of Human Papillomavirus among Women Attending a Well Woman Clinic. *Sex Transm Infect* 2003; 79:320–322.

Weinstock H, Berman S, Cates W, Jr. Sexually Transmitted Diseases among American Youth: Incidence and Prevalence Estimates, 2000. *Perspect Sex Reprod Health.* 2004;36:6–10.

Zimet GD, Perkins SM, Sturm LA, Bair RM, Juliar BE, Mays RM. Predictors of STI Vaccine Acceptability among Parents and Their Adolescent Children. *J Adolesc Health* 2005 September;37(3):179–186.

Zimet GD. Improving Adolescent Health: Focus on HPV Vaccine Acceptance. *J Adolesc Health* 2005 December;37(6) Supplement 1:S17–S23.

Chapter 10: Vaccines on the Global Front: Unique Challenges and Opportunities

AIDS Vaccine Advocacy Coalition. The Emerging Adolescent Agenda: HPV Vaccine, AIDS Prevention Research, and the New Opportunities for Reaching the Young People of the World, from the 2006 AVAC Report, AIDS Vaccines: The Next Frontiers. http://www.avac.org/pdf/reports/2006_Report/AVAC_ch3.pdf. Accessed April 2008.

Agurto I, Arrossi S, White S, et al. Involving the Community in Cervical Cancer Prevention Programs. *Int J Gynaecol Obstet* 2005, 89, S38–S45.

Carter M. HPV Vaccine Shows Good Efficacy, but How Valuable Will It Be in 'Real World' Settings? May 11, 2007. Found online at http://aidsmap.com/. Accessed March 2008.

Culture, a Barrier to Pap Tests for Mexican Women. *Reuters Health Information.* April 6, 2007. Available online at http://www.reuters.com/article/health News/idUSSIB65795920070406?feedType=RSS. Accessed May 2008.

Denny L. The Prevention of Cervical Cancer in Developing Countries. BJOG. *Int J Obst Gyn.* 2005;112(9):1204–1212.

Denny L, Kuhn L, de Souza M, Pollack AE, Dupree W, Wright TC. Screen-and-Treat Approaches for Cervical Cancer Prevention in Low Resource Settings. *JAMA.* 2005 November 2;294:2173–2181.

Denny L, Quinn M, Sankaranarayanan R. Screening for Cervical Cancer in Developing Countries. *Vaccine.* 2006;24(S3):S71–S77.

Denny L., Sankaranarayanan R: Secondary Prevention of Cervical Cancer *Int J Obstet Gynecol* 2006;94(S1):S65–S70.

Fisher K, Bass E. Advocacy, Information and Communication: Engaging Stakeholders at All Levels to Prepare for the Introduction of HPV Vaccines. This background paper was prepared by the AIDS Vaccine Advocacy Coalition (AVAC) for the December 12-13, 2006 meeting: "Stop Cervical Cancer: Accelerating Global Access HPV Vaccines.

Freeman HP. Cancer in the Socioeconomically Disadvantaged. *CA Cancer J Clin* 1989; 39: 266–288.

Freeman HP. Cancer in the Economically Disadvantaged. *Cancer* 1989; 64(Suppl 1): 324–334; discussion 342–325.

Freeman HP. Commentary on the Meaning of Race in Science and Society. *Cancer Epidemiol Biomarkers Prev* 2003; 12: 232S–236S.

Goldie SJ, Kohli M, Grima D, et al. Projected Clinical Benefits and Cost-Effectiveness of a Human Papillomavirus 16/18 Vaccine. *Journal of the National Cancer Institute* 2004;96(8):604–614.

Goldie SJ, Kuhn L, Denny L, Pollack A, Wright TC Jr. Policy Analysis of Cervical Cancer Screening Strategies in Low-Resource Settings. Clinical Benefits and Cost Effectiveness. *JAMA.* 2001, 285: 3107–3115.

Grey N, Sener S. Reducing the Global Cancer Burden; *Patient Care.* March 1,2006. Available online at http://www.hospitalmanagement.net/features/feature 648/. Accessed May 2008.

Jayant K, Rao RS, Nene BM, Dale PS. Improved Stage at Diagnosis of Cervical Cancer with Increased Cancer Awareness in a Rural Indian Population. *Int J Cancer.* 1995;63:161–163.

Koutsky LA, Patridge JM. Genital Human Papillomavirus Infection in Men. *The Lancet Infectious Diseases.* 2006;6(1):21–31.

Leiman G. "Project Screen Soweto"—A Planned Cervical Screening Program in a High-Risk Population. *South African Medical Journal* 1987;2: 61–68.

MacKenzie D. Will Cancer Vaccine Get to All Women. Newscientist.com; April 18, 2005. Available online at http://www.newscientist.com/channel/sex/mg18624954.500-will-cancer-vaccine-get-to-all-women.html. Accessed June 2008.

Megevand E, Denny L, Dehaeck K, Soeters R, Bloch B. Acetic Acid Visualization of the Cervix: An Alternative to Cytologic Screening.*Obstet Gynecol* 1996;88: 383–386.

Munoz N, Bosch FX, Castellsagué X, et al. Against Which Human Papillomavirus Type Shall We Vaccinate and Screen? The International Perspective. *Int J Cancer* 2004. 111: 278–285.

Pan American Health Organization. Human Papillomavirus Vaccines—A New Tool for Cervical cancer Prevention. http://www.paho.org/. Accessed April 2008.

Parkin DM. The Global Health Burden of Infection—Associated Cancers in the Year 2002. *Int J Cancer* 2006;118(12):3030–3044.

Pollack AE. HPV Vaccines: An Overview. Assuring Access to Vaccines that Prevent Cervical Cancer; Stop Cervical Cancer: Accelerating Global Access to HPV Vaccines. December 12–13, 2006, London. Available online at http://www.rho.org/files/StopCxCa_access_2006.pdf. Accessed May 2008.

Pollack AE, Balkin MS, Edouard L, Cutts F, Broutet N. Assuring Access to Human Papillomavirus Vaccines. A Reproductive Health Perspective Bulletin.

Program for Appropriate Technology in Health (PATH). Planning Appropriate Cervical Cancer Prevention Program, 2nd ed. 2000. http://www.path.org/files/cxca-planning-appro-prog-guide.pdf

Royal Thai College of Obstetricians and Gynaecologists (RTCOG) and the JHPIEGO Corporation Cervical Cancer Prevention Group. Safety, Acceptability, and Feasibility of a Single-Visit Approach to Cervical-Cancer Prevention in Rural Thailand: A Demonstration Project. *Lancet.* 2003;361(9360):814–820.

Sankaranarayanan R, Esmy P, Rajkumar R, et al. Effect of Visual Screening on Cervical Cancer Incidence and Mortality in Tamil Nadu, India: a Cluster-Randomised Trial. *Lancet* 2007;370(9585):398–406.

Sankaranarayanan R. Overview of Cervical Cancer in the Developing World Cancer. *Int J Gynaecol Obstet* 2006;95(S1):S205–S210.

Sankaranarayanan R, Budukh AM, Rajkumar R. Effective Screening Programmes for Cervical Cancer in Low- and Middle-Income Developing Countries.*Bull World Health Organ.* [online]. 2001;79(10): 954–962. http://whqlibdoc.who.int/bulletin/2001/issue10/79(10)954-962.pdf. Accessed April 2008.

Sankaranarayanan R, Rajkumar R, Esmy PO, et al. Effectiveness, Safety and Acceptability of 'See and Treat' with Cryotherapy by Nurses in a Cervical Screening Study in India. *Br J Cancer* 2007;96;738–744.

Sankaranarayanan R, Rajkumar R, Theresa R, et al. Initial Results from a Randomised Trial of Cervical Visual Screening in Rural South India. *Int J Cancer* 2004;109:461–67.

Sankaranarayanan R, Thara S, Sharma A, et al. for the Multicentre Study Group on Cervical Cancer Early Detection in India. Accuracy of Conventional Cytology: Results from a Multicentre Screening Study in INDIA. *J Med Screen* 2004;11 (34):77–84.

Sankaranarayanan R, Wesley R, Somanathan T, et al. Visual Inspection of the Uterine Cervix after the Application of Acetic Acid in the Detection of Cervical Carcinoma and its Precursors. *Cancer* 1998;83(10):2150–2156.

Sankaranarayanan R, Shyamalakumary B, Wesley R, Sreedevi Amma N, Parkin DM, Nair MK. Visual Inspection with Acetic Acid in the Early Detection of Cervical Cancer and Precursors. *Int J Cancer* 1999;80:161–163.

Schiffman M, Castle PE. The Promise of Global Cervical-Cancer Prevention; *NEJM.* 2005;353(20):2101–2104.

Suba EJ, Murphy SK, Donnelly AD, Furia LM, Huynh MLD, Raab SS. Systems Analysis of Real-World Obstacles to Successful Cervical Cancer Prevention in Developing Countries. *Am J Public Health.* 2006;96(3):480–487.

Tsu VD, Pollack AE. Preventing Cervical Cancer in Low-Resource Settings: How Far Have We Come and What Does the Future Hold? *Int J Obstet Gynecol* 2005;89:S55–S59.

Ward E, Jemal A, Cokkinides V, Singh GK, Cardinez C, Ghafoor A, Thun M. Cancer Disparities by Race/Ethnicity and Socioeconomic Status. *CA Cancer J Clin* 2004;54(2):78–93.

World Health Organization (WHO). Global Strategy for the Prevention and Control of Sexually Transmitted Infections: 2006–2015. Geneva: World Health Organization; 2006. http://whqlibdoc.who.int/hq/2006/WHO_RHR_06.10 _eng.pdf. Accessed April 2008.

World Health Organization (WHO). Preparing for the Introduction of HPV Vaccines: Policy and Programme Guidance for Countries. Geneva: World Health Organization; 2006.

INDEX

AAFP (American Association of Family Practice), 103–4
AAP (American Academy of Pediatrics), 104, 120
ABC (abstinence, being faithful, and condom use), 185
ablative procedures, 61
abnormal lesions of the cervix. *See* cervical dysplasia
abstinence, 4–5, 7, 8, 30, 87, 94, 152–53, 185
adenocarcinoma *in situ*, 101
adolescents. *See* teenagers
adrenaline, 32
Advisory Committee on Immunization Practices (ACIP), 1–2, 4. *See also* Centers for Disease Control and Prevention
Adyar Cancer Institute, 180
Africa, 174, 176. *See also specific countries by name*
African Americans: anal cancer rates, 56; cervical cancer deaths and incidence rates, 37, 66; HPV prevalence among males, 121; penile cancer rates, 126; public education about HPV infections, 168
age: of first intercourse as HPV risk factor, 30; HPV DNA testing, 43–44; of HPV infected people, 17, 18; HPV vaccines approved for, 102–3;

recommended age for HPV vaccinations, xi, 8, 102–3, 138–39, 142, 150–51, 160; as risk factor, 33; of women with cervical cancer, 33, 42, 44
AIDS. *See* HIV/AIDS
AIN (anal intraepithelial neoplasia), 127
AIS (Cervical Aden Carcinoma in situ), 158
Alaska, 9, 66
alcohol and drug abuse, 32–33, 88, 123–25, 152
allergies to vaccine components, 110, 160
aluminum, 163
Alzheimer's dementia, 163
American Academy of Pediatrics (AAP), 104, 120
American Association of Family Practice (AAFP), 103–4
American Association of Obstetricians and Gynecologists, 61
American Cancer Society: anal cancer estimates, 56; on cervical cancer death rates, 18, 32, 36–37, 39, 65, 156; HPV DNA recommendations, 44; on HPV-related throat cancer, 124; on HPV vaccines, 73; Pap test guidelines, 40, 41
American College of Pathology, 42

ABOUT THE AUTHOR

SHOBHA S. KRISHNAN, M.D., is Staff Physician at Columbia University's Barnard College Health Services. A board certified gynecologist and family practice physician, she has also worked as a surveillance physician for the federal Centers for Disease Control and Prevention. Prior to joining Barnard, she was in private practice for 10 years. In addition, Dr. Krishnan has worked as a physician at the Institute on Aging and as Chief Resident in the Family Practice Department at St. Vincent Hospital, Indianapolis. Any comments or questions about this book can be emailed to hpvvaccinebook@gmail.com.